10-Minute
STRENGTH TRAINING EXERCISES FOR SENIORS

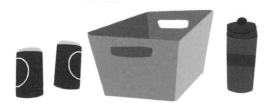

10-Minute STRENGTH TRAINING EXERCISES FOR SENIORS

Exercises and Routines to Build
Muscle, Balance, and Stamina

ED DEBOO, PT

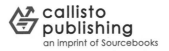

callisto
publishing
an imprint of Sourcebooks

I would like to thank my amazing wife, Elizabeth, whose unwavering love and support inspire me daily.

Published by Callisto Publishing LLC C/O Sourcebooks LLC
P.O. Box 4410, Naperville, Illinois 60567-4410
(630) 961-3900
callistopublishing.com

Printed and bound in China.
OGP 10 9 8 7 6 5 4 3 2 1

Contents

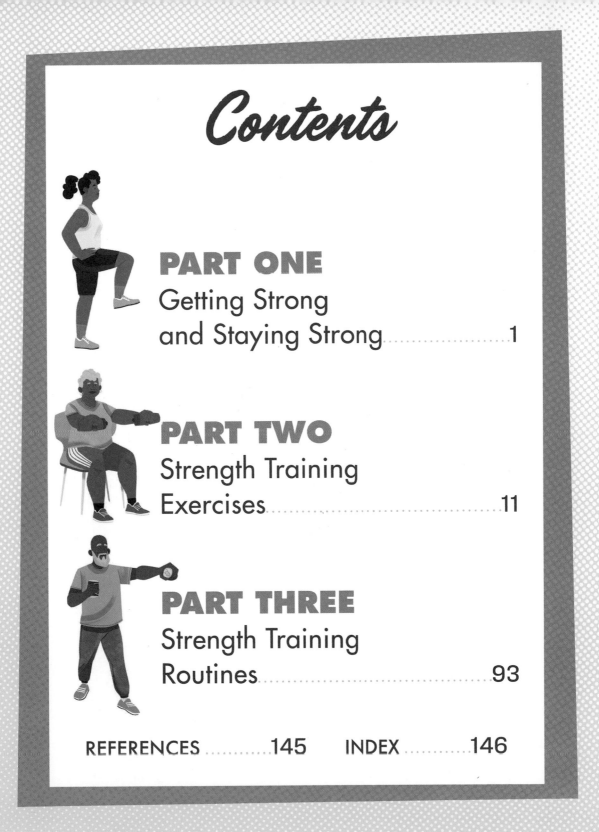

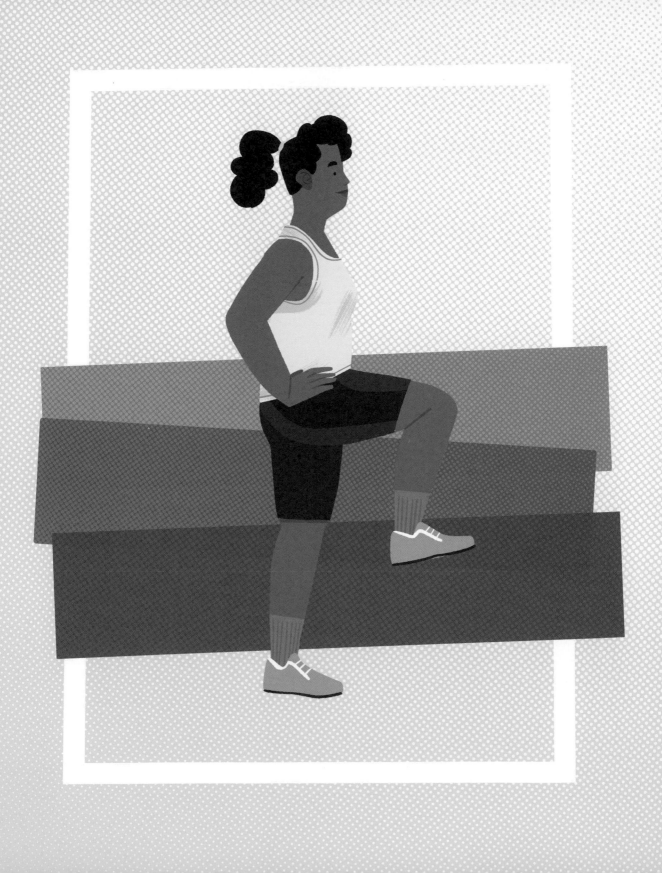

PART ONE

GETTING STRONG AND STAYING STRONG

AS A PHYSICAL THERAPIST with over twenty-nine years of clinical experience, I firmly believe that strength training is the most important factor in enhancing the quality of life for older adults. As you age, your muscles may weaken, and your bones become less dense, which can lead to falls and a loss of independence.

However, with just ten minutes of strength training per day, you can maintain and build your muscle mass, improve your bone density, and reduce the risk of chronic diseases. No matter your physical condition, you can get stronger.

It's truly amazing to see my clients grow stronger, increase their mobility, and become more confident in their abilities. It enables them to maintain their independence and enjoy life to the fullest. Tennis, anyone?

I will cover the numerous benefits of strength training and provide you with invaluable insights on how to safely embark on a strengthening program, including proper warm-up, cooldown, and injury prevention tips. In addition, I will guide you through forty diverse strengthening exercises for your entire body, with clear instructions on how to make each exercise more challenging or easier to accommodate your fitness level. Then, using a combination of the exercises, I have outlined twenty-five different routines to keep your exercises fresh! Let this book enhance your health and help you lead a more active and fulfilling life.

WHAT IS STRENGTH TRAINING?

Strength training is a series of resistance exercises that target different muscle groups to increase strength and muscular endurance. Its numerous benefits for seniors include improved independence, better balance and mobility, increased bone density, and a reduced risk of chronic disease. Despite the benefits, myths limit many seniors from this life-enriching practice. Let's look at why these myths are wrong.

Older adults cannot get stronger.

Not true! Numerous studies, including one by Dr. Kieran Reid and colleagues, demonstrated improved mobility, strength, and better balance in seniors with consistent strength training. They compared strength training programs, using both lighter and heavier loads, and determined that both routines created significant strength and power improvements. Seniors can get stronger, add muscle mass, and improve their functional ability, regardless of age and current level of health, even with lighter resistance.

Strength training is dangerous for seniors and can cause injury.

On the contrary, strength training can protect joints, reduce inflammation, and help you prevent injuries. By increasing muscle strength and stability, there is a reduction of stress and load on the joints. Additionally, strength training stimulates the release of cytokines, our body's natural anti-inflammatory agents, leading to decreased inflammation and aiding in injury prevention. With the proper instructions and intensity, strength-training exercises are very safe and effective.

Seniors should only lift light weights.

Lifting heavier weights is safe. The key lies, however, in understanding one's limits. Strength training requires a slow and progressive approach. Start with lighter weights and gradually increase the resistance as you become comfortable and confident in your abilities. Focus on your form and listen to your body's signals, such as muscle discomfort and fatigue.

Seniors need to go to the gym or use specialized equipment to strength train.

Household items such as soup cans, laundry baskets, and gallon jugs can be effectively used to gain strength. Bodyweight exercises such as squats, lunges, and push-ups can be easily modified based on strength levels.

By finding enjoyable and engaging exercises, setting achievable goals, and tracking progress, strength training can be both rewarding and enjoyable!

THE BENEFITS OF STRENGTH TRAINING

Strength training is a powerful tool for transforming your body and mind. It builds muscles, strengthens bones, improves balance and flexibility, enhances metabolism, promotes weight management, and reduces the risk of chronic diseases. Enhancing your strength makes it much easier to do daily activities such as carrying groceries, getting on the floor, working in the yard, and climbing stairs.

Muscular Strength and Endurance

Muscular strength refers to the maximum force a muscle can generate, whereas muscular endurance refers to the ability of muscles to sustain repetitive contractions over an extended period. Activities such as gardening that involve both muscular strength and endurance become effortless and fun as you get stronger.

Bone Density

Strength training places positive "stress" on bones, which stimulates the body to increase bone density. Bone density decreases with age, leading to an increased risk of fractures. Stronger bones improve quality of life by reducing the risk of fractures and make impact activities such as sports and hiking safer.

Movement and Mobility

Strength training increases muscle mass and improves bone density and joint stability. This results in better coordination, balance, and flexibility—all of which reduce the risk of falls and injuries. Strength training also helps improve posture by strengthening the muscles that support the spine, shoulders, and neck.

Metabolic Health

Measures of metabolic health include healthy levels of cholesterol and normal blood pressure. Strength training improves metabolic health by reducing inflammation, reducing your risk of cardiovascular disease, and promoting fat loss. As your metabolic health improves, you will sleep better and have more energy.

Immunity

Strength training has been shown to increase the production of immune cells. A stronger immune system means that you may be less likely to get sick and have shorter recovery times if you do. Further benefits of improved mood and increased energy enhance your immune system function.

Joint Health

Strengthening the muscles that support the joints leads to reduced joint pain and increased joint mobility. As your strength increases, the subsequent stress on your joints lessens. This can help prevent and manage conditions such as osteoarthritis and improve overall physical function and quality of life.

Balance and Fall Prevention

Strength training helps improve balance and reduce the risk of falling by increasing lower-body strength and stability, improving coordination and reaction time, and increasing proprioception (your body's internal sense of position, movement, and balance). Improved proprioception allows you to regain your balance and become more sure-footed when walking on uneven or slippery surfaces.

Aches and Pains

Imagine waking up with less pain and stiffness, ready to conquer the day. Strengthening exercises release endorphins, your body's natural painkillers that can help alleviate joint pain, stiffness, and aches. Strengthening the muscles around the joints helps reduce joint pressure and strain as well.

Mental Health

In addition to the pain-relieving effects, endorphins also induce a sense of well-being, improving your mood. Exercise also releases serotonin, a neurotransmitter, that helps regulate mood and sleep. This makes strength training a great drug-free way to boost your self-esteem, reduce symptoms of depression, and enhance your brain health.

Live Longer and Stronger

Strength training offers a multitude of benefits that can enhance your life and promote longevity. By improving muscular endurance, bone density, mobility, balance, and supporting mental health, while also boosting immunity and reducing aches and pains, you can empower yourself to maintain independence and enjoy a stronger, more fulfilling life journey.

GETTING STARTED SAFELY

It's never too late to get started, even if you're brand-new to weight training. If you are returning to exercise after a break, it is important to take a gradual approach, beginning with light weights and focusing on proper form to reduce the risk of injury and ensure better results. Prioritizing consistency over intensity for the first two to four weeks will help build a baseline level of strength and give your body a chance to acclimate to the new "stress."

Muscle soreness typically occurs twenty-four to forty-eight hours after a workout and is a normal response to exercise. It is characterized by pain, stiffness, and tenderness. Although uncomfortable, muscle soreness is a sign that your muscles are adapting to the stress of use and getting stronger. However, it is important to distinguish between post-exercise soreness and pain that may be a sign of injury. Normal soreness should improve within a few days, whereas pain that persists may require you to rest and recover before your next workout.

Every exercise can be modified to provide both easier and more challenging options, ensuring that individuals of all fitness levels and abilities can participate and progress according to their specific needs and goals.

Get Medical Clearance

As a physical therapist, I have decades of experience in recommending exercises to strengthen people's bodies, and I always prioritize safety to reduce the risk of injury. However, the information and exercises in this book should not be used in place of the advice of your healthcare provider.

It is vital to consult your healthcare provider before starting any exercise program, especially if you have existing health conditions. Even after receiving clearance to exercise, watch for warning signs that require you to stop exercising immediately—such as joint pain or swelling, heart palpitations, dizziness, or chest pain—and seek further medical evaluation.

HOW TO USE THIS BOOK

Are you ready to feel better, get stronger, and have some fun? Let's dive in and take action! With forty comprehensive exercises targeting every part of your body and twenty-five dynamic routines, you'll be fully prepared for any adventure or activity you have in mind. Remember, the key to success lies in making these exercises and routines your own, incorporating them into your daily life, and creating empowering habits that will propel you toward your fitness goals. Consistency is the key!

Stretching, Warming Up, and Cooling Down

It is essential when exercising to briefly warm up beforehand and to then cool down from a workout with light activity. Whereas stretching involves lengthening muscles, strengthening involves placing the muscle under tension with resistance to gain strength. Warming up before the strengthening process helps increase muscle temperature and flexibility, optimizing performance and reducing the risk of injury. Cooling down after your workout promotes recovery, enhancing the overall effectiveness of the strengthening process.

Before exercising, perform a five-minute warm-up, such as marching in place or climbing stairs, to increase blood flow and prepare your body to exercise. After exercising, do a five-minute cooldown, such as slow walking or light stretching, to slowly allow your body to return to its resting state. Doing so can help reduce muscle soreness and reduce your risk of injury. Additional examples of warm-up and cooldown exercises can be found in part 2.

Exercises

The book explains forty distinct strengthening exercises that target various upper-body muscles, such as those in the chest, shoulders, arms, and back, as well as lower-body muscles of the hips, knees, and ankles. With the flexibility to choose exercises in any order, you can tailor your workout based on fitness goals and areas of need. Within each exercise, you will find helpful reminders to ensure safe execution and maximize the benefits derived from each movement. In addition, modifications allow for adjustments in intensity to accommodate different fitness levels by describing ways to make each exercise easier or more challenging.

The exercises in this book are osteoporosis-safe because they prioritize maintaining a neutral spine, which reduces the risk of compression fractures in individuals with osteoporosis. By avoiding excessive spinal flexion (forward bending) or rotation, these exercises minimize the strain on the spine and promote safe movements that protect against potential injuries.

Routines

Using the forty upper- and lower-body strengthening exercises, I have created twenty-five unique, ten-minute exercise routines, each offering targeted benefits. Each routine consists of four exercises, incorporating essential rest intervals to optimize strengthening gains.

From functional tasks such as gardening and hiking to specific body parts, such as hips and shoulders, and even focusing on fall prevention, bone density, and cardiac fitness, there's a routine for everyone. With options like Total Body Tune-Up (page 95), Balance Booster (page 101), Joint Juice Jive (page 135), and Knee Pain Knockout (page 143), you can enjoy a different workout each day. Once familiar with the exercises, feel free to personalize your routine by selecting your favorite four exercises.

Make Strength Training a Lifestyle

When it comes to establishing an exercise routine as part of your lifestyle, it's easy to start with great motivation and excitement, only to fall off the wagon. However, it's never too late to embrace a healthy lifestyle. Daily reflection on your progress can provide you with the motivation and determination to keep exercising.

Starting small and focusing on short-term fitness goals can also help you stay motivated and build confidence. Though the routines are only ten minutes long, you will begin to experience significant rewards.

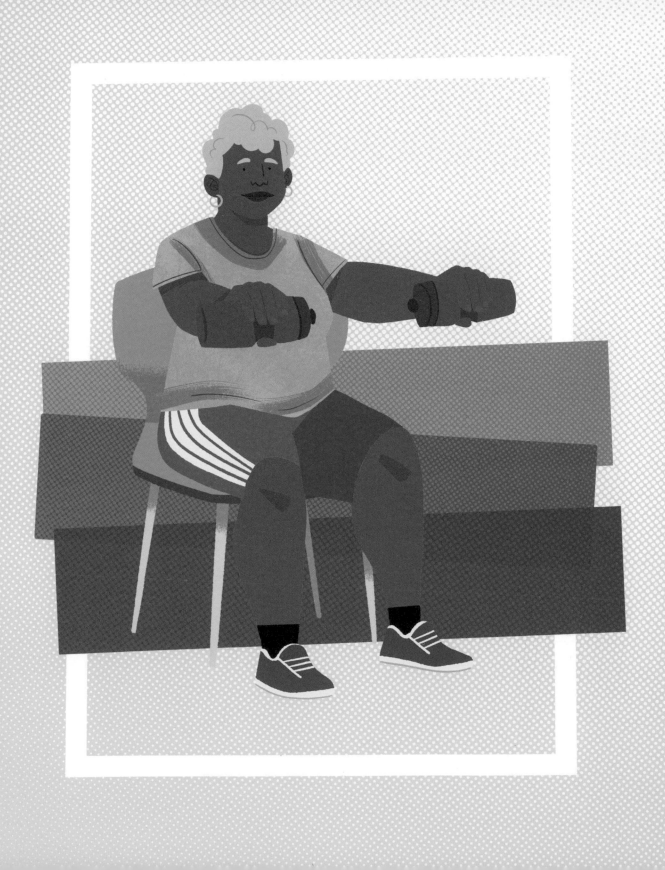

PART TWO

STRENGTH TRAINING
EXERCISES

GET READY TO MOVE AND GROOVE! I will help you stay strong, active, and healthy with just ten minutes of exercise per day!

These strengthening exercises are designed to be safe yet challenging, accessible to all fitness levels, and most importantly, fun. With a focus on the chest, shoulders, arms, and back muscles, the upper-body exercises will have you feeling strong and toned. The lower-body exercises, on the other hand, target the muscles of the hip, knee, and ankle, improving your balance and stability, and making your body ready for anything. Keep in mind that a neutral spine entails keeping your back straight within its natural alignment, without slouching or arching, to protect your spine and prevent strain or injury; whereas an engaged core means gently pulling your belly button in toward your spine while keeping your back straight.

Each exercise will have clear illustrations of proper form and technique, the names of the targeted muscles, reminders to keep you safe, and modifications to make each exercise either harder or easier.

Staying active and strong is key to living your best life, no matter what your age. Whether you're new to fitness or a seasoned pro, you'll find something to love in this series. So, let's get started and make every day a happy and healthy one!

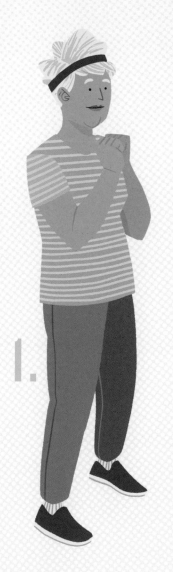

1.

REMEMBER

As you squat, your knees should not extend past your toes, keeping your feet flat on the floor. Some weight on your heels will help. If you experience knee pain as you squat lower, start with a smaller range of motion, and then increase the depth as you become stronger.

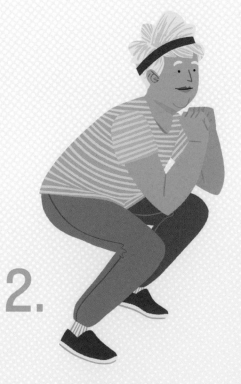

2.

SQUATS

TARGETED MUSCLE GROUPS: Calves, Glutes, Hamstrings, Quadriceps

Ah, the Squat—a personal favorite of mine! Every time you get up from a chair, you are doing a Squat. Squats are a great exercise that strengthens the major muscles in the lower body. The benefits of Squats include enhanced balance and bone density, and stronger legs will make walking, climbing stairs, and even jumping easier.

INSTRUCTIONS

1. Stand with your feet shoulder-width apart, toes slightly pointed outward. Keep your back straight and engage your core. Clasp your hands together in front of your body.

2. Bend your knees and drive your hips back as if you were sitting in a chair, keeping your weight on your heels. Lower yourself until your thighs are parallel to the floor. Pause for a moment, then drive your hips forward and stand back up.

3. Inhale as you go down and exhale as you stand up. Complete 8 to 12 repetitions for 1 set. Do 2 or 3 sets total with 30 to 60 seconds of rest in between sets.

Easy Modification: Use a bench or a chair for support. Stand in front of the bench or chair with your feet shoulder-width apart and slowly lower yourself until you touch the seat with your butt. Then push back up to the starting position.

Challenging Modification: Add resistance by holding a heavy object, such as a full jug of water or a backpack full of books, close to your chest. You can also hold the squat position for 2 or 3 seconds before standing back up.

> **REMEMBER**
>
> Stand up tall and engage your core by visualizing that you are drawing your belly button into your spine. Keep your head straight to help with balance and make sure to breathe throughout the exercise. This is a good warm-up exercise.

THE STORK

TARGETED MUSCLE GROUPS: Core Muscles, Gluteus Medius, Piriformis

The muscles of your hips can become weak when you don't engage in lateral movements as often as you once did. Lateral movements are all about moving sideways, such as shuffling across the court during pickleball. This simple but very effective exercise is a great way to build up endurance in your core and hips, and improve your balance to keep you rock steady on your feet.

INSTRUCTIONS

1. Stand sideways next to the wall with your shoulder just a few inches away. Bend the knee closest to the wall so it is just below your hip and push it into the wall with moderate force.

2. Hold this contraction for 10 to 15 seconds and repeat 2 or 3 times on each side. That is 1 set. Complete 2 or 3 sets on each hip and rest for 30 to 60 seconds in between sets.

Easy Modification: If it's hard to balance during this exercise, use a chair for support. Also, start with a lighter contraction and shorter hold times until you can improve your endurance.

Challenging Modification: Use a small ankle weight or push harder into the wall. Increasing the hold times to 20 to 30 seconds will also make it more challenging.

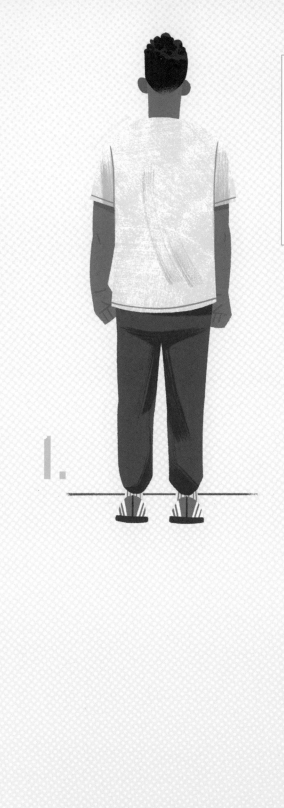

1.

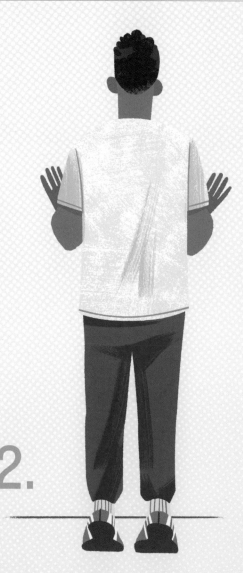

2.

HEEL RAISES

TARGETED MUSCLE GROUPS: Gastrocnemius, Soleus

Lower leg swelling and poor circulation are common conditions that often leading to cramping, swelling, and cold feet. Not only will Heel Raises help improve lower leg circulation, but you can also hit the trails and embark on adventurous hikes, navigating rugged terrain with ease and confidence.

INSTRUCTIONS

1. Stand facing a wall, about an arm's length away.

2. Using your hands on the wall for balance, slowly lift your heels off the floor, pause, and slowly come back down.

3. Complete 8 to 12 repetitions for 1 set. Do 2 or 3 sets total with 30 to 60 seconds of rest in between sets.

Easy Modification: If lifting your heels is difficult, use the support of a kitchen counter or desk to allow you to leverage your arms for help. In addition, start either by sitting in a chair or by not lifting your heels very far off the ground.

Challenging Modification: Balance on one leg first and do single-leg heel lifts. You can also hold a small weight in one hand or hold the contracted position for 3 to 5 seconds.

WALL SITS

TARGETED MUSCLE GROUPS: Glutes, Hamstrings, Quadriceps

Wall Sits help improve lower-body strength, which is used in various sports such as trail running, hiking, and soccer. In addition, improving lower leg strength is critical to help you get up from the floor, climb stairs, and get up out of a chair. Wall Sits are an excellent exercise to improve muscular endurance and strength and reduce knee and hip pain.

INSTRUCTIONS

1. Start by leaning against a wall, with your feet about 12 inches away. Slowly slide down until your thighs are parallel to the floor. Keep your back flat against the wall for the entire exercise and your hands clasped together at your waist. Then push back up to a standing position.

2. Complete 8 to 12 repetitions for 1 set. Do 2 or 3 sets total with 30 to 60 seconds of rest in between sets.

Easy Modification: With slightly bent knees, do "mini" squats and slowly slide down farther as you become stronger. Stand with a wider stance if balance is an issue. You can also put your arms by your sides for support.

Challenging Modification: Hold the sitting position for 5 to 10 seconds before you come back up to a standing position. You can also hold a small weight in each hand to add more resistance.

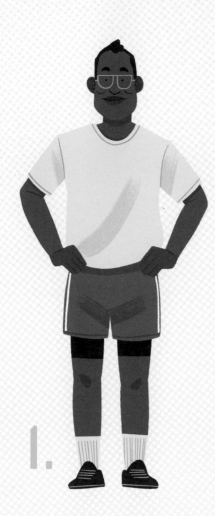

1.

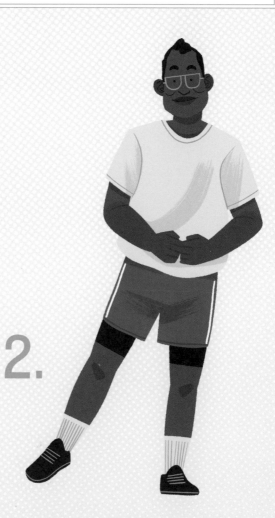

2.

STANDING HIP ABDUCTION

TARGETED MUSCLE GROUP: Gluteus Medius

This exercise does a great job of strengthening your hips and improving your balance and stability. A strong gluteus medius helps alleviate hip and lower back pain and stabilizes your hips not only for walking, but for higher-level activities such as running and jumping.

INSTRUCTIONS

1. Stand with your feet shoulder-width apart, engage your core, and place your hands on your hips.

2. Lift your right leg out to the side as far as you can while keeping your hips level. Keep your left leg straight and your toes pointing forward. You may fold your hands together in front of your body if this is more comfortable.

3. Hold this position for 1 to 3 seconds and then lower your leg back down to the starting position. Complete 8 to 12 repetitions for 1 set. Do 2 or 3 sets total with 30 to 60 seconds of rest in between sets.

Easy Modification: Start by lifting your leg only a few inches to the side and/or use a chair for balance and support.

Challenging Modification: Hold the abducted position for 5 to 10 seconds before you bring your leg back down to your side. In addition, use a small ankle weight around your ankles.

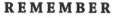

1.

2.

MOUNTAIN CLIMBERS

TARGETED MUSCLE GROUPS:
Abdominals, Calves, Deltoids, Glutes, Hamstrings, Triceps

Mountain Climbers are one of my favorite exercises to boost speed and balance and prevent falls by improving your reaction times. Improving reaction time helps you regain your balance by increasing the speed with which you can move your legs. This exercise engages multiple muscle groups and gets you ready to hit the trails!

INSTRUCTIONS

1. Place your hands on the kitchen counter or the back of a couch, below your shoulders. Your hands should be shoulder-width apart. Step back so your body is at a slight angle to the counter or couch. Your back should be straight from your head to your heels.

2. With your right foot on the ground, lift your left knee toward your chest. Quickly switch your stance by bringing your left leg down and bringing your right knee up toward your chest. Continue alternating legs as quickly as you can while maintaining your awareness on a strong, stable core. Keep your back in a straight line from head to heels.

3. Complete 8 to 12 repetitions for 1 set. Do 2 or 3 sets total with 30 to 60 seconds of rest in between sets.

Easy Modification: Start slowly and focus on your form. You can also perform the exercise with your hands elevated on a higher surface to reduce the amount of weight on your arms and shoulders.

Challenging Modification: Perform the exercise on the floor instead, in a push-up position, and increase the number of repetitions and speed. You can add a push-up after each repetition.

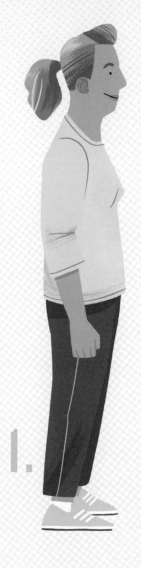

1.

REMEMBER
Maintain your body in a straight line, and don't bend forward as you move your leg behind you. Keep your toes pointed straight and avoid rotating your hip outward. To avoid overloading your lower back muscles, it's important to keep your movements controlled and avoid swinging your leg.

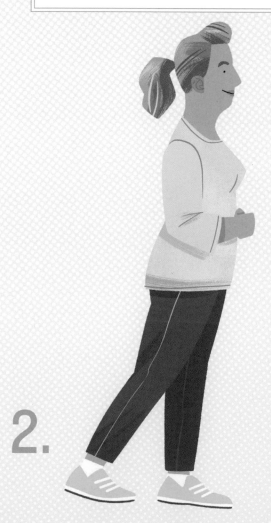

2.

STANDING HIP EXTENSION

TARGETED MUSCLE GROUPS:

Gluteus Maximus, Hamstrings, Lumbar Spine Erectors

This exercise not only strengthens and tones your glutes but also improves your balance and stability, helping you dominate activities such as kicking a soccer ball, powering up a hill during a hike, and getting in and out of a car. As a bonus, you will also strengthen your lower back muscles, helping your posture and reducing lower back pain.

INSTRUCTIONS

1. Stand sideways, with your left shoulder next to a wall. Rest your left hand on the wall for balance and support.

2. Engage your core, shift your weight onto your left leg, and lift your right leg off the ground behind you, keeping your knee as straight as you can, your toes pointed forward and foot flat.

3. Complete the movement slowly for 8 to 12 repetitions on the same leg, then switch sides. Do a total of 2 or 3 sets on each leg with 30 to 60 seconds of rest in between sets.

Easy Modification: Reduce the number of repetitions and decrease how far back you move your leg. If balance is an issue, perform the exercise while facing your kitchen counter and use both hands for support and stability.

Challenging Modification: Increase the number of repetitions, add a hold of 2 or 3 seconds when your leg is behind your back, or add small ankle weights. For a greater challenge, forgo the wall support.

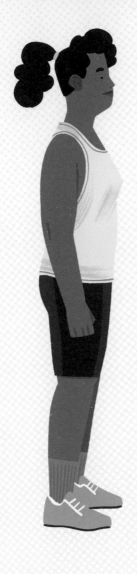

1.

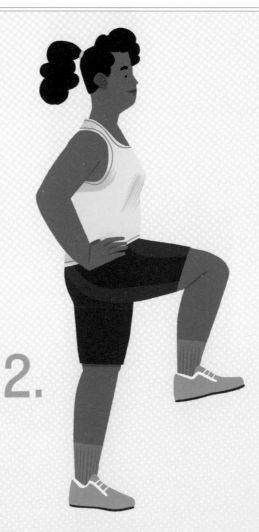

2.

HIGH KNEES

TARGETED MUSCLE GROUPS:
Core Muscles, Glutes, Hamstrings, Psoas, Quadriceps

Ready to run faster and feel stronger on your feet? This is a great exercise to improve your lower-body strength, flexibility, balance, and speed and enhance your cardiovascular health. It also improves your coordination by requiring you to lift one leg at a time while maintaining stability on the other. This exercise can also be used for a warm-up.

INSTRUCTIONS

1. Stand with your left shoulder next to a wall. Rest your left hand on the wall for balance and support.

2. With your right hand on your hips, lift your right knee toward your chest as high as you can comfortably while keeping your left foot firmly on the ground. Lower your right leg and repeat with your left leg.

3. Continue alternating legs at a comfortable pace for 10 to 15 repetitions for 2 or 3 sets with 30 to 60 seconds of rest in between sets.

Easy Modification: Reduce the number of repetitions, slow down your pace, and decrease how far up you bring your knees. If balance is an issue, perform the exercise in between two heavy chairs and use both hands for support and stability, or perform the exercise sitting.

Challenging Modification: Increase your speed and the number of repetitions or use small ankle weights. Also, not using the wall for support will challenge your balance even further.

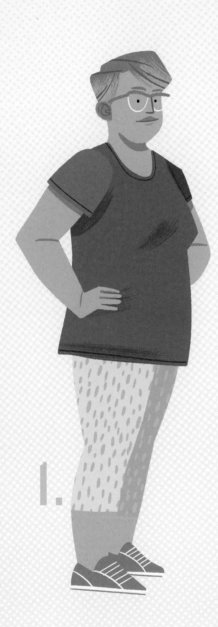

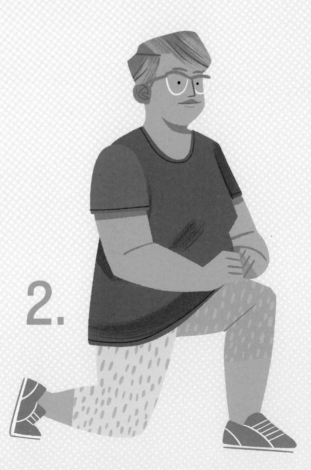

1.

2.

FRONT LUNGES

TARGETED MUSCLE GROUPS:
Calves, Core Muscles, Glutes, Hamstrings, Quadriceps

Front Lunges are a very functional exercise that will improve your balance, flexibility, and lower-body strength. Getting up and down from the floor can become challenging, but this exercise will allow you to safely get onto the floor as well as pick up items without stressing your lower back.

INSTRUCTIONS

1. Stand with your feet shoulder-width apart with your core engaged and your hands on your hips.

2. Keeping your back as straight as you can, take a step forward with your left leg and lower your body until your front knee is bent to about 90 degrees. Your back knee should hover just above the ground. Push through your left heel and return to the starting position. If needed for support, you can move your hands to the front of your body, above your knee.

3. Complete 8 to 12 repetitions on each side for 1 set. Do 2 or 3 sets total with 30 to 60 seconds of rest in between sets.

Easy Modification: Decrease the depth of the lunge or hold on to a chair for support. If additional support is needed, stand in between two sturdy, heavy chairs and use both arms for support and balance as needed.

Challenging Modification: Hold small weights in each hand, hold the forward lunge position for 3 to 5 seconds, or increase the depth of the lunge.

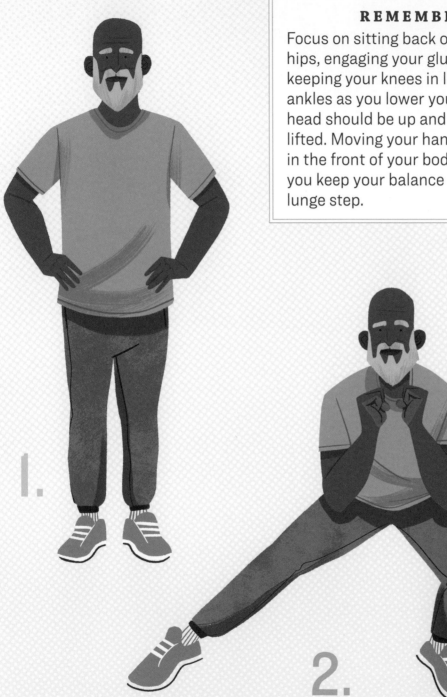

REMEMBER

Focus on sitting back onto your hips, engaging your glutes, and keeping your knees in line with your ankles as you lower your body. Your head should be up and your chest lifted. Moving your hands together in the front of your body will help you keep your balance during the lunge step.

1.

2.

SIDE LUNGES

TARGETED MUSCLE GROUPS:
Adductors, Calves, Core Muscles, Glutes, Hamstrings, Quadriceps

Pivoting on a tennis court or doing Warrior Pose in yoga both require strong hip muscles. The Side Lunge is a multi-joint movement that targets several important muscles involved in side-to-side balance and stability. By incorporating Side Lunges into your routine, you are enhancing lateral stability and building powerful inner and outer thighs.

INSTRUCTIONS

1. Stand with your feet shoulder-width apart with your core engaged and your hands on your hips.

2. With your left foot, take a big step to your left and bend your left knee, keeping the other leg straight. Lower your body as far as you can or until your thigh is parallel to the ground. Push through your left heel and return to the starting position. You can clasp your hands together in front of your body for balance during the lunge.

3. Complete 8 to 12 repetitions for 1 set on each side. Do 2 or 3 sets total with 30 to 60 seconds of rest in between sets.

Easy Modification: Decrease the depth of the lunge and hold on to a chair for support and balance.

Challenging Modification: Hold a small weight in your hands, hold the forward lunge position for 3 to 5 seconds, or increase the depth of the lunge.

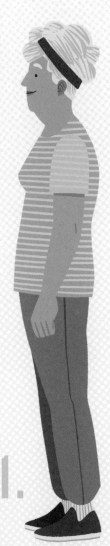

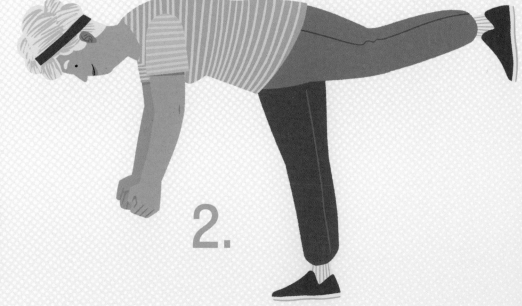

1.

2.

SINGLE-LEG DEADLIFT

TARGETED MUSCLE GROUPS:

Calves, Core Muscles, Glutes, Hamstrings, Lower Back, Quadriceps

Ready to nail that Tree Pose in yoga? The Single-Leg Deadlift is an excellent exercise to improve your balance, strength, and flexibility in one movement. With practice, you will feel steadier on your feet, gain flexibility in your hamstrings, and improve your balance for biking or any other sport or activity you want to try!

INSTRUCTIONS

1. Stand with a slight bend in your knees, with your weight on your right foot. Engage your core.

2. Keeping your back straight, slowly bend forward at your hips, extending your right leg behind you for balance. Keep your arms straight and in front of your body to help with balance. While maintaining good form, lower your body toward the floor as far as you can go. Then return to the standing position.

3. Complete 8 to 12 repetitions for 1 set on each leg. Do 2 or 3 sets per leg with 30 to 60 seconds of rest in between sets.

Easy Modification: Use a chair for support and balance. You can also limit how far you hinge forward.

Challenging Modification: Hold small weights in your hands or increase the depth of the hinge.

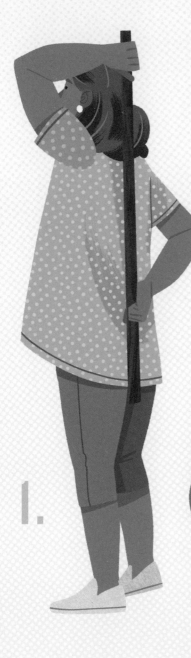

1.

2.

> ### REMEMBER
>
> It's important to maintain a straight spine during the exercise. During the movement, if you lose either the contact point of your tailbone or the back of your head with the broom handle, make sure you are hinging at the hips and not rounding your lower back. Although your knees are slightly bent, don't bend your knees farther during the exercise; instead focus on hinging at the hips.

HIP HINGE

TARGETED MUSCLE GROUPS:
Calves, Core Muscles, Glutes, Hamstrings, Lower Back, Quadriceps

Due to the repeated forward bending, sports such as golf and tennis can be hard on the lower back, leading to pain. This is an excellent exercise to reduce lower back pain during daily activities that involve forward bending. In addition to sports, loading the dishwasher, doing laundry, and cooking are a few examples of when you can Hip Hinge to protect your lower back.

INSTRUCTIONS

1. Stand with your feet shoulder-width apart and a slight bend in your knees. Hold a broom behind your back, with one end contacting your tailbone and the other touching the back of your head. The broom is used as a tool to help you maintain a straight back during the forward bend while hinging at the hips.

2. Keeping your core engaged, hinge at your hips and lower your upper body until you feel a stretch in your hamstrings. Keep the broom in contact with the back of your head and tailbone throughout the exercise. You will often be limited by tightness in your hamstrings at the end of the movement.

3. Complete 8 to 12 repetitions for 1 set. Do 2 or 3 sets total with 30 to 60 seconds of rest in between sets.

Easy Modification: Until you master the movement, you can limit how far you hinge forward.

Challenging Modification: Once the hip hinge becomes second nature, you no longer need the broom. Instead, hold small weights in your hands and increase the depth of the hinge.

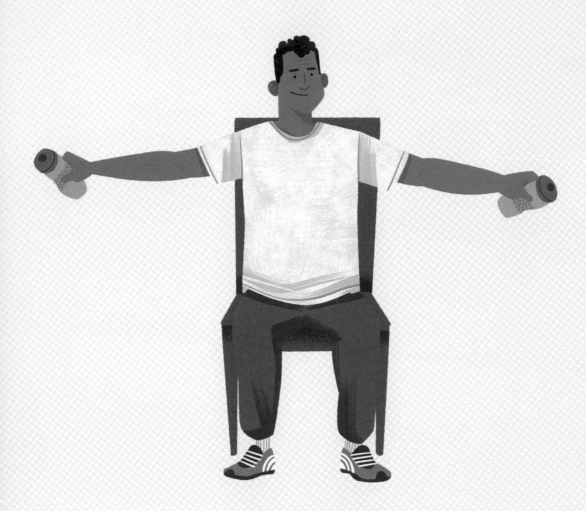

REMEMBER

Keep your shoulders back and down throughout the movement to avoid unnecessary strain on your neck. Bring your arms a bit forward if you experience shoulder pain. Don't raise your arms higher than shoulder height, as this may irritate your rotator cuff muscles.

SHOULDER LATERAL RAISES

TARGETED MUSCLE GROUPS: Lateral Deltoids, Rotator Cuff, Upper Trapezius

Get ready to tackle life's demands head-on with strong, injury-resistant shoulders and a confident posture. This exercise does a great job helping improve shoulder strength and endurance. Increased strength of your shoulders will help make activities such as lifting groceries into the trunk of your car or watering your plants much easier.

INSTRUCTIONS

1. Sit in a chair with your feet flat on the ground and hold a light weight in each hand, palms facing inward and arms resting at your sides.

2. Slowly raise your arms out to the sides until they reach shoulder height, then lower them back down to your sides.

3. Complete 8 to 12 repetitions for 1 set. Do 2 or 3 sets total with 30 to 60 seconds of rest in between sets.

Easy Modification: Use lighter weights or no weights at all. Reduce the range of motion by not lifting your arms as high and taking longer rest periods between sets.

Challenging Modification: Use heavier weights, hold the contracted position for 3 to 5 seconds before you bring your arms back down, or slow down the movement to increase your muscular time under tension.

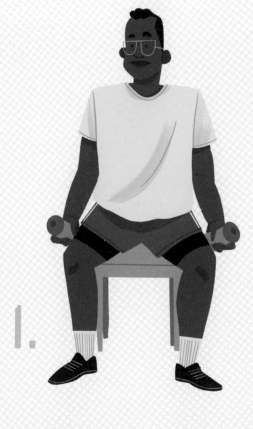

1.

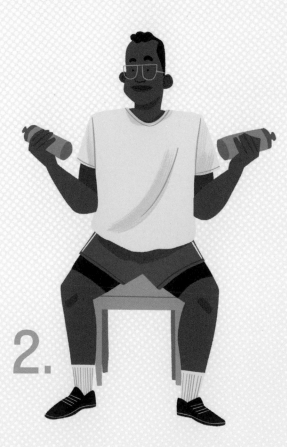

2.

BICEP CURLS

TARGETED MUSCLE GROUPS: Biceps, Forearms, Grip Strength, Wrists

Bicep Curls will make your arms and wrists stronger and improve your grip strength. Greater arm strength makes everyday activities, such as carrying groceries or pulling weeds in the garden, much easier. You can also take to the water and master paddleboarding with your newfound bicep strength.

INSTRUCTIONS

1. Prepare two small weights, such as water bottles, before starting. Sit up tall with your feet shoulder-width apart and hold a weight in each hand.

2. Slowly lift the weights toward your shoulders by bending your elbows, keeping your elbows close to your sides. When your elbows are fully bent, pause for 1 second, then slowly return to the starting position.

3. Complete 8 to 12 repetitions for 1 set. Do 2 or 3 sets total with 30 to 60 seconds of rest in between sets.

Easy Modification: Start with lighter weights, such as a can of soup in each hand. You can also lean back in a chair to support your back until you gain core strength.

Challenging Modification: Use heavier weights, such as a 5-pound dumbbell, in each hand and perform the exercise standing up. You can try standing on one leg to work your balance as well as arm strength.

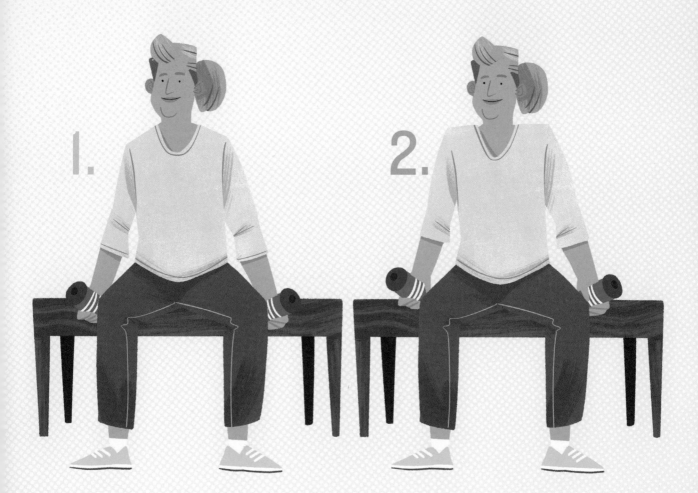

1.

2.

REMEMBER
Focus on the proper form by sitting up tall, keeping your shoulder blades squeezed together to improve your posture, and breathing throughout the exercise.

SHOULDER SHRUGS

TARGETED MUSCLE GROUPS: Deltoids, Neck, Upper Trapezius

Upper trapezius muscles are where many of us carry stress, making them sore and painful. Shoulder Shrugs to the rescue! This simple but very effective exercise helps reduce neck and shoulder tension, improve posture, and increase shoulder mobility. Shoulder shrugs can be done anytime and anywhere, making them an excellent exercise to incorporate into your daily routine or use for a warm-up.

INSTRUCTIONS

1. Sit with your feet shoulder-width apart and your arms hanging down by your sides. Have a small weight in each hand.

2. Keeping your elbows straight, slowly shrug both shoulders up toward your ears, hold for 1 to 2 seconds, then lower them back down to the starting position.

3. Complete 8 to 12 repetitions for 1 set. Do 2 or 3 sets total with 30 to 60 seconds of rest in between sets.

Easy Modification: Start without any weights, using just the weight of your arms. Also, limit your range of motion by not shrugging too high.

Challenging Modification: Hold heavier weights in your hands and pause for 3 to 5 seconds at the top. To improve your balance, do the exercise standing up or even while balancing on one leg.

1.

2.

SHOULDER FRONT RAISES

TARGETED MUSCLE GROUPS: Anterior Deltoids, Biceps, Forearms, Trapezius

Is that gallon of milk getting heavier to lift? Stronger shoulders improve your ability to reach and grab objects from high shelves or cabinets, making everyday tasks easier, and adding speed to your golf swing. In addition, having stronger shoulders also protects you from injury and preserves your joints, making you more resilient.

INSTRUCTIONS

1. Sit up straight in a chair, engaging your core, with your feet flat on the floor. With your arms at your sides, hold a small weight, such as a water bottle, in each hand.

2. Slowly raise both arms straight out in front of you until they are at shoulder height, keeping your palms facing down. Hold for 1 to 2 seconds, then slowly return to the starting position.

3. Complete 8 to 12 repetitions for 1 set. Do 2 or 3 sets total with 30 to 60 seconds of rest in between sets.

Easy Modification: Use lighter or no weights and limit how high you bring your arms. You can also do this exercise one arm at a time.

Challenging Modification: Use heavier weights and hold the contracted position for 3 to 5 seconds before lowering your arms to your sides. To challenge your balance, you can stand up or even balance on one leg during the exercise.

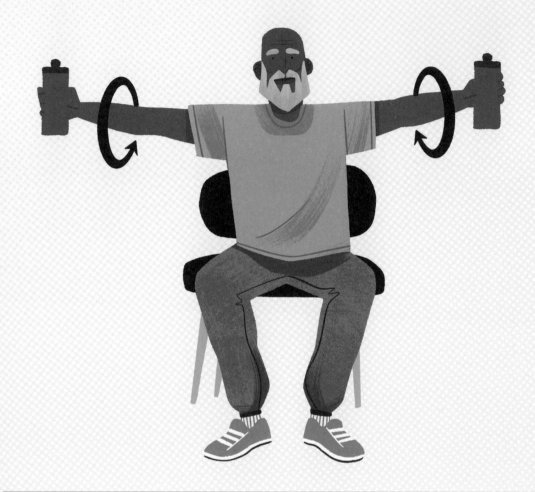

REMEMBER

Keep your shoulder blades back and down throughout the exercise to maintain proper form and prevent shoulder strain. Focus on keeping your arms straight and maintaining a controlled pace throughout the exercise.

ARM CIRCLES

TARGETED MUSCLE GROUPS: Lateral Deltoid, Rotator Cuff, Trapezius

Unlock the power in your shoulders with this exercise that improves shoulder mobility, flexibility, and muscular endurance, making repetitive tasks, such as swimming, tai chi, and dribbling a basketball, easier and less fatiguing.

INSTRUCTIONS

1. Sit in a chair with good posture, your feet flat on the floor, and your core engaged. With a light weight in each hand, extend your arms straight out to your sides at shoulder height. Slowly rotate your arms in small circles, gradually making them larger in a comfortable range of motion.

2. Complete 8 to 12 revolutions for 1 set. Make sure to change directions and keep your palms facing forward. Repeat 2 or 3 sets total with 30 to 60 seconds of rest in between sets.

Easy Modification: Use lighter or no weights and limit how high you bring your arms. Make smaller circles and slow down your pace with longer rest intervals between sets.

Challenging Modification: Use heavier weights, increase the number of revolutions per set, and gradually increase your arm speed. You can also perform the exercise standing up to work on balance.

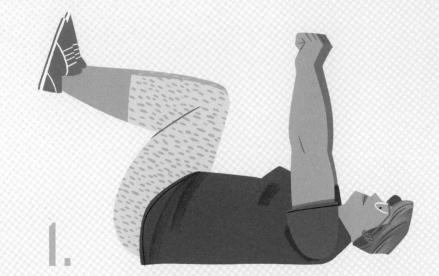

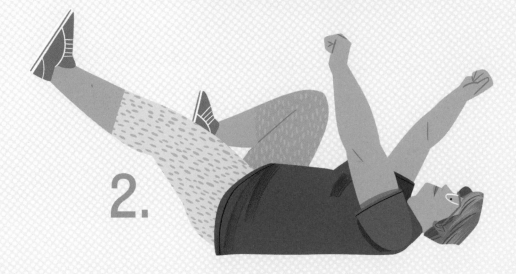

REMEMBER

Keep your lower back in contact with the floor throughout the entire exercise to prevent lower back strain and maximize the effectiveness of the exercise. If you have trouble keeping your lower back flat, you may need to reduce the angle of your arm and leg lowering until your core becomes stronger.

DEAD BUG

TARGETED MUSCLE GROUPS:

Obliques, Psoas, Quadriceps, Rectus Abdominis, Transverse Abdominis

Imagine bending and twisting your spine with ease, without pain. Well, you can with this exercise. Strong core muscles help protect our spine and reduce the pain of arthritis. This exercise targets the deep core muscles that play critical roles in stabilizing your spine, improving your balance, and maintaining good posture.

INSTRUCTIONS

1. Lie on your back with arms extended straight up toward the ceiling and your knees bent at a 90-degree angle so your shins are parallel to the ground.

2. Slowly lower your right arm and left leg simultaneously toward the floor while keeping your lower back in contact with the floor. Then return to the starting position and repeat on the opposite side by lowering your left arm and right leg simultaneously to the floor.

3. Complete 8 to 10 repetitions with each arm for 1 set. Repeat Do 2 or 3 sets total and rest for 30 to 60 seconds in between sets.

Easy Modification: Reduce the range of motion by not lowering your arms as far toward the floor and instead of holding your leg up in the air, touch your toes to the ground at an angle.

Challenging Modification: Lower your arms and legs closer to the floor and hold the extended position for 3 to 5 seconds before bringing them back to the starting position. In addition, use small ankle and wrist weights to add resistance.

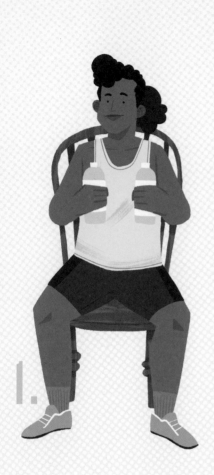

> **REMEMBER**
> Focus on keeping your elbows close to your sides throughout the exercise to target the rotator cuff muscles. If your shoulder is tight, you may not be able to rotate your arm very much. However, don't worry; take it as far as you can without pain, and eventually your range of motion should increase.

1.

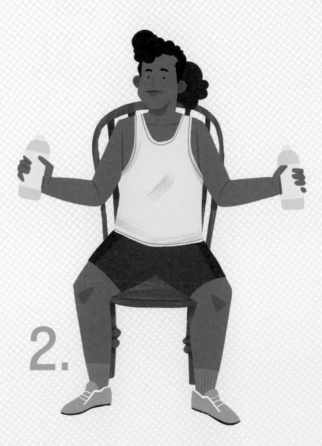

2.

SHOULDER BLADE SQUEEZES

TARGETED MUSCLE GROUPS: Rhomboids, Rotator Cuff, Trapezius

Various yoga poses and Pilates exercises involve arm balances and overhead positions that rely heavily on shoulder stability and control. A strong rotator cuff provides the necessary support to hold these positions with proper alignment, preventing injury to the shoulder joint. Focusing on strengthening these important muscles protects your shoulders and keeps you doing what you love.

INSTRUCTIONS

1. Sit in a chair with good posture, your feet flat on the floor, and your core engaged. With a light weight in each hand, bend your elbows to a 90-degree angle.

2. Keeping your elbows close to your body, rotate your shoulders outward so your forearms move away from your body. Pause for 1 to 2 seconds while squeezing your shoulder blades together, then return to the starting position.

3. Complete 8 to 12 repetitions for 1 set. Do 2 or 3 sets total with 30 to 60 seconds of rest in between sets.

Easy Modification: Use lighter weights or no weights at all to start. Also, limit the amount of outward rotation of your shoulders until your mobility improves.

Challenging Modification: Use heavier weights, increase the number of repetitions per set, or perform the exercise standing up with your feet close together to work on balance.

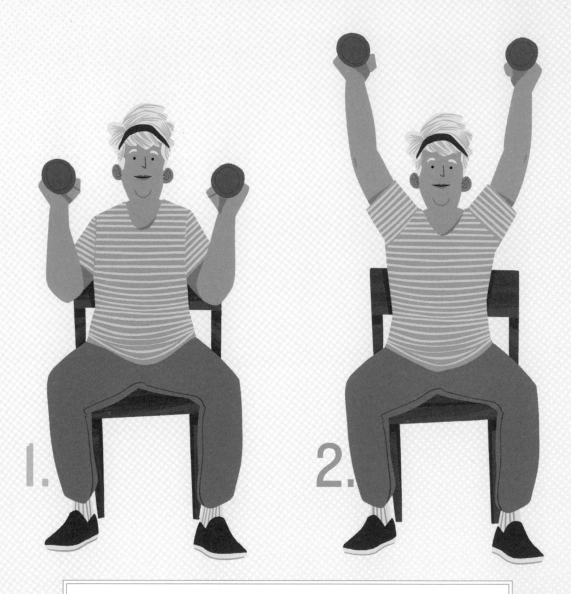

1.

2.

REMEMBER

Start with light weights and gradually increase as you get stronger. Avoid arching your lower back as you lift the weights overhead. Bring your elbows closer together if you experience shoulder discomfort. Exhale as you push the weights up and inhale as you lower them down.

OVERHEAD PRESS

TARGETED MUSCLE GROUPS: Deltoids, Pectoralis, Trapezius, Triceps

Putting your luggage in an overhead bin when traveling requires strong shoulders and core muscles. The Overhead Press is a great way to improve upper-body strength and endurance. Activities like putting away groceries and reaching into the top kitchen cabinet become easier and effortless.

INSTRUCTIONS

1. Sit in a chair with good posture, your feet flat on the floor, and your core engaged. With a light weight in each hand, bend your elbows and raise the weights to your shoulders.

2. Push the weights above your head until your arms are fully extended. Pause for 1 to 2 seconds, then lower the weights back down to your shoulders.

3. Complete 8 to 12 repetitions for 1 set. Do 2 or 3 sets total with 30 to 60 seconds of rest in between sets.

Easy Modification: Use lighter or no weights and limit how high you bring your arms. You can also do fewer repetitions until your strength increases.

Challenging Modification: Use heavier weights and increase the number of repetitions per set. You can also perform the exercise standing up with a narrow base of support to work on balance.

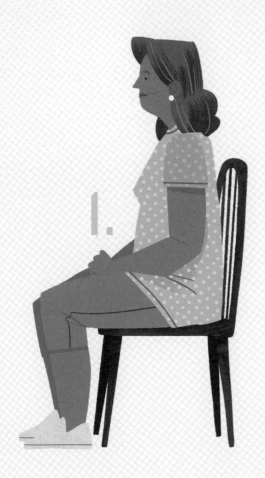

SEATED KNEE EXTENSION

TARGETED MUSCLE GROUP: Quadriceps

This exercise can help you effortlessly climb stairs, hike uphill without fatigue, and play pickleball with agility and stability. Seated knee extensions are a great way to add power and stability to your legs by increasing the strength of your quadriceps muscles.

INSTRUCTIONS

1. Sit in a chair with good posture, your feet flat on the floor and your core engaged.

2. Slowly extend your left leg with your toe pointed up until your knee is as straight as possible. Hold for 1 to 2 seconds, then slowly lower your leg back to the floor. Repeat the same movement on the other leg.

3. Complete 8 to 12 repetitions for 1 set on each leg. Do 2 or 3 sets total per leg with 30 to 60 seconds of rest in between sets.

Easy Modification: Use lighter weights or decrease the range of motion by not fully extending your knee at the top of the movement. Also, do fewer repetitions when first starting.

Challenging Modification: Use heavier weights on your ankles, increase the number of repetitions per set, and increase the hold time to 3 to 5 seconds when your leg is fully extended.

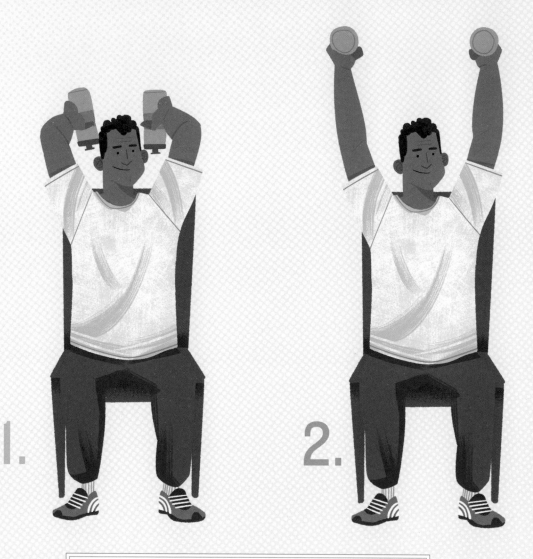

1.

2.

TRICEP PRESS

TARGETED MUSCLE GROUP: Triceps

Target and strengthen the muscles located at the back of your upper arm with this exercise. Strong triceps provide essential support to the shoulders and upper back, contributing to improved posture. Say hello to toned arms as you effortlessly lift heavy suitcases and nail those push-up repetitions.

INSTRUCTIONS

1. Sit in a chair with your back straight and your core engaged. Hold a light weight in each hand. Raise your arms above your head, bend your elbows to about 90 degrees, and slowly lower the weights behind your head.

2. Lift both weights toward the ceiling, straightening your arms. Pause for 1 to 2 seconds, then slowly bend your elbows and lower the weight behind your head.

3. Complete 8 to 12 repetitions for 1 set. Do 2 or 3 sets total with 30 to 60 seconds of rest in between sets.

Easy Modification: Use lighter weights or decrease the range of motion by not fully extending your arms at the top of the movement. You can also do fewer repetitions when first starting or hold one weight with both hands.

Challenging Modification: Use heavier weights, increase the number of repetitions per set, and increase the hold time to 3 to 5 seconds when your arms are fully extended over your head.

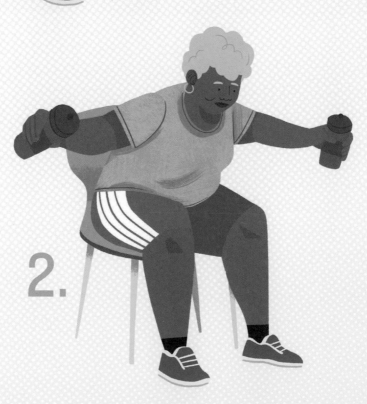

1.

REMEMBER

Avoid rounding your back as you lean forward. Instead, focus on hinging at your hips and maintaining a straight back. You may need to practice hinging at the hips first to make sure you understand the movement before you add weight and the arm movements. Looking in a mirror to determine proper posture may also be helpful.

2.

REVERSE FLIES

TARGETED MUSCLE GROUPS:
Lower Back, Posterior Deltoid, Rhomboids, Rotator Cuff

Are your shoulders starting to round forward? This is a result of weakness in your upper back muscles. This exercise is an excellent way to help you stand up straighter, improve your posture, and gain upper-body strength. Better posture can also help alleviate pain and discomfort in your neck and shoulders.

INSTRUCTIONS

1. Sit in a chair with your feet flat on the ground and your core engaged. Hold a light weight in each hand with your palms facing each other and your elbows bent to a 90-degree angle. Keeping your back straight, lean forward from your hips.

2. Slowly lift your arms out to the sides, keeping your elbows bent, and squeeze your shoulder blades together. Hold for 1 to 3 seconds, then lower the weights to the starting position.

3. Complete 8 to 12 repetitions for 1 set. Do 2 or 3 sets total with 30 to 60 seconds of rest in between sets.

Easy Modification: Use lighter weights or no weights at all to start and reduce the hold time when your arms are out to your sides. Also, limit how far out you bring your arms.

Challenging Modification: Use heavier weights, increase the number of repetitions per set, and increase the hold time to 3 to 5 seconds when your arms are out to your sides.

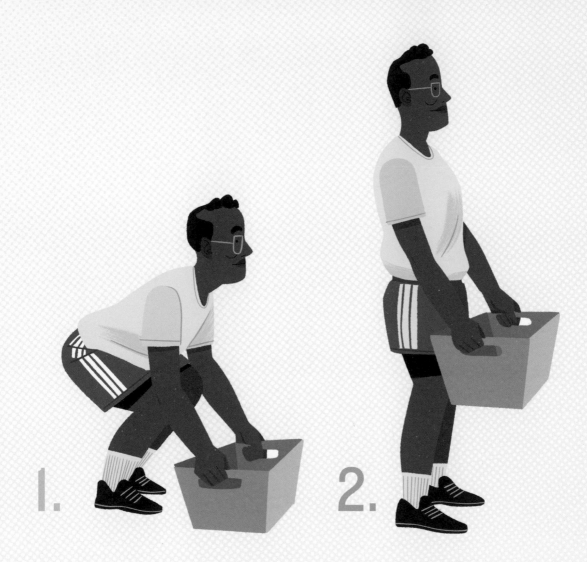

1.

2.

REMEMBER

Use a firm laundry basket with good handles. Avoid rounding your back as you squat. Focus on hinging at your hips and keep your knees aligned with your ankles. Your arms should be straight during the entirety of the exercise. If your back starts to fatigue, stop the exercise and check your form.

DEADLIFT

TARGETED MUSCLE GROUPS: Glutes, Hamstrings, Latissimus Dorsi, Lower Back

Laundry day just got easier! Deadlifts are one of my favorite exercises and probably one of the most functional exercises to help you stay strong in both your arms and legs. It is a multi-joint exercise that improves strength in your core, lower back, and legs to improve balance, stability, and posture.

INSTRUCTIONS

1. Stand with your feet shoulder-width apart with a laundry basket in front of you. Keeping your back straight, drive your hips back, squat down, and grab the handles of the laundry basket with both hands.

2. Keeping your back straight and core engaged, slowly lift the basket by pushing through your heels until you are standing straight up. Pause, then lower the basket back to the floor. That is 1 repetition.

3. Complete 8 to 12 repetitions for 1 set. Do 2 or 3 sets total with 30 to 60 seconds of rest in between sets.

Easy Modification: Place an empty laundry basket on a raised surface. This allows you to work on your form and strength before practicing lifting it from the floor.

Challenging Modification: Place more weight in the laundry basket, increase the number of repetitions per set, and increase the hold time to 3 to 5 seconds when the basket is off the floor.

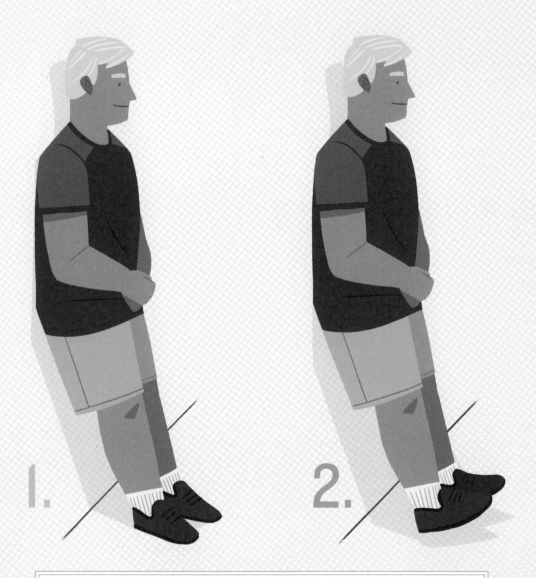

REMEMBER

Perform this exercise on a nonslip surface so your feet won't slide away from you. Do not lock your knees; instead, have a very slight bend in them until you feel your thigh muscles tighten. Keep your shoulders relaxed and avoid leaning forward. Your back should stay flat on the wall.

TOE LIFTS

TARGETED MUSCLE GROUP: Tibialis Anterior

If the muscles in your feet and shins become weak, you can be at risk of developing a shuffling type of walking pattern, leading to an unsteady gait and increased risk of falls. Say goodbye to shin splints. This exercise strengthens the muscle that runs up the front of your shin, supporting your knees and ankles while helping you walk more safely.

INSTRUCTIONS

1. Stand with your back leaning against a wall and your feet out in front of you, shoulder-width apart, keeping them about 6 to 8 inches away from the wall. Have good balance and feel steady on your feet.

2. Slowly lift your toes off the floor, shifting your weight onto your heels. Hold for 5 seconds, then slowly lower your toes to the floor.

3. Complete 8 to 12 repetitions for 1 set. Do 2 or 3 sets total with 30 to 60 seconds of rest in between sets.

Easy Modification: Do not hold the toe-lifted position. Instead, pause momentarily and then lower your toes to the floor. Use a chair for balance or perform the exercise while sitting until you get stronger.

Challenging Modification: Use small weights in your hands, increase the number of repetitions per set, and increase the hold time from 5 seconds to 10 seconds when your toes are lifted.

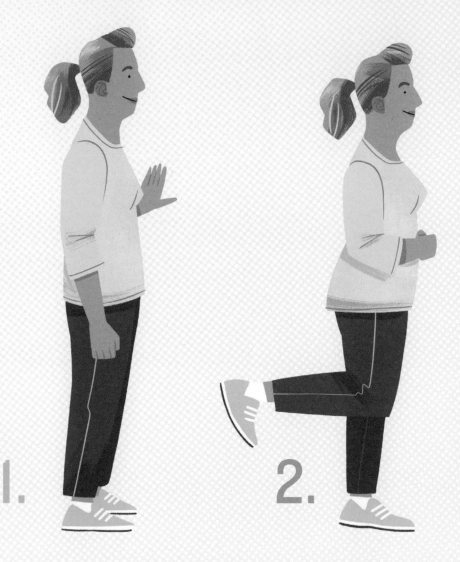

1.

2.

REMEMBER

Avoid using momentum to lift your heel toward your buttocks. Focus on contracting the muscles in the back of your thigh in a slow, controlled fashion. If you have had a knee injury, you may not be able to bend your knee very far. However, moving through your available range of motion will help you build strength.

STANDING LEG CURLS

TARGETED MUSCLE GROUP: Hamstrings

This exercise improves your lower-body strength and endurance and helps protect your knees. Stronger hamstrings provide you the power to kick a soccer ball and ride a bike, and they also support your lower back while bending, helping maintain proper alignment and reduce the risk of injury.

INSTRUCTIONS

1. Stand with your left side next to a wall and place your left hand on the wall for support. Engage your core and shift your weight to your left leg.

2. Contract the muscles of your left leg for added stability, then slowly bend your right knee, lifting your heel toward your buttocks. Pause for 2 or 3 seconds, then return your leg down to the starting position. Avoid leaning forward when bending your knee.

3. Complete 8 to 12 repetitions for 1 set. Do 2 or 3 sets total with 30 to 60 seconds of rest in between sets.

Easy Modification: Do not hold your heel in the contracted position. Instead, momentarily pause, then return it to the floor. Also, limit your knee bend initially until you get stronger, or use a kitchen countertop for balance instead of the wall.

Challenging Modification: Use ankle weights, increase the number of repetitions per set, and increase the hold time to 3 to 5 seconds when your knee is bent.

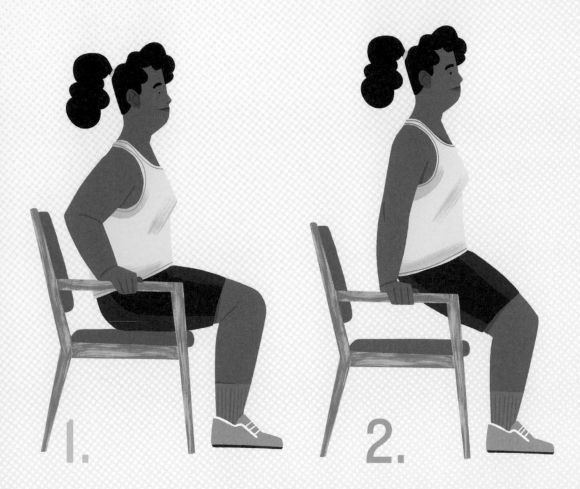

REMEMBER

Keep your elbows close to your sides throughout the exercise to engage your triceps more effectively and protect your shoulders. Keep your back straight, but if you do need to lean forward, remember to hinge your hips.

CHAIR TRICEP DIPS

TARGETED MUSCLE GROUPS: Deltoid, Pectoralis, Triceps

Ready to tone your upper arms and get stronger? These seated tricep dips are a great exercise to improve shoulder, chest, and arm strength. The benefits extend beyond aesthetics, as stronger triceps assist in daily activities, such as lifting heavy groceries, pushing yourself up from a seated position, and pushing open heavy doors.

INSTRUCTIONS

1. Sit toward the front of a sturdy chair with armrests. Hold on to the armrest with both hands in a tight grip.

2. Slowly lift your body up from the chair using your arms. Pause for 1 to 2 seconds, then slowly lower your body back to the chair.

3. Complete 8 to 12 repetitions for 1 set. Do 2 or 3 sets total with 30 to 60 seconds of rest in between sets.

Easy Modification: Do not hold the contracted position. Instead, momentarily pause, then return to the chair. Additionally, use a cushion on your chair to make it easier to lift your upper body and limit how high you go.

Challenging Modification: Place a small weight on your lap, increase the number of repetitions per set, or increase the hold time to 3 to 5 seconds before returning to your chair. To challenge your core muscles, allow one leg to hover above the floor before you lift your upper body.

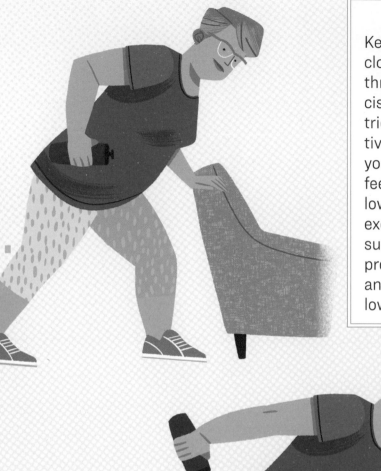

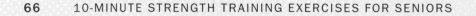

TRICEP KICKBACKS

TARGETED MUSCLE GROUPS: Posterior Deltoid, Triceps

Add muscle mass and power to your upper arms with these kick-backs. If activities such as standing up from a low chair and putting items on the top shelf of a closet are sometimes difficult due to the weakness of your arms, increasing the strength of your triceps will make these activities much easier and safer.

INSTRUCTIONS

1. Stand next to a table or chair in a staggered stance with your left leg in front and your right leg behind you. Using your left hand for balance and keeping your back straight, hinge forward from the hips. Hold a light weight in your right hand with your elbow bent at a 90-degree angle. Lift your elbow until it is behind your shoulder and parallel to the floor.

2. Slowly straighten your arm, keeping your elbow close to your side. Pause for 1 to 2 seconds with your elbow fully extended, then slowly bend your elbow to the starting position.

3. Complete 8 to 12 repetitions for 1 set. Do 2 or 3 sets total with 30 to 60 seconds of rest in between sets.

Easy Modification: Use lighter weights and do not hold the con-tracted position. Instead, momentarily pause, then slowly bend your elbow, returning to the starting position.

Challenging Modification: Use heavier weights and hold the con-tracted position for 3 to 5 seconds before you bend your elbow. To challenge your balance, do the exercise without holding on to a chair for support. You can also do both arms at the same time.

WALL PUSH-UPS

TARGETED MUSCLE GROUPS: Deltoids, Pectoralis, Triceps

Wall Push-Ups are a multi-joint exercise that transforms your chest, shoulders, and arms into powerhouses. This simple exercise will help you push open heavy doors and even make handling a full cart during your next grocery run much easier.

INSTRUCTIONS

1. Find a wall with enough space to freely bend your arms during the exercise. Stand up straight and place your palms on the wall, slightly lower than shoulder height.

2. Bend your elbows as you lean in toward the wall. Your elbows will be at about a 45-degree angle away from your body. When you get close to the wall, pause for a second, then push back to the starting position.

3. Complete 8 to 12 repetitions for 1 set. Do 2 or 3 sets total with 30 to 60 seconds of rest in between sets.

Easy Modification: Stand closer to the wall and limit your range of motion so you are not bending your elbows as far.

Challenging Modification: Stand farther back from the wall. As you become stronger, you may want to use a lower surface, such as the kitchen counter, to make your muscles work harder.

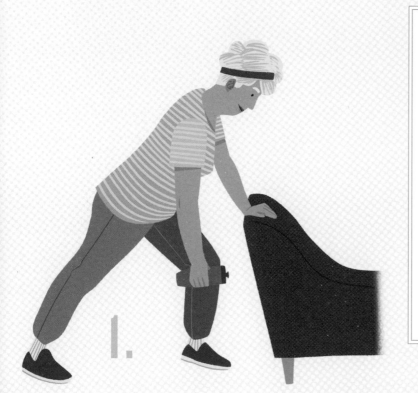

REMEMBER
Keep your elbows close to your sides through-out the exercise. If you feel a strain on your lower back, stop the exercise and make sure you are hinging properly from the hips and not rounding your lower back. Avoid looking up, focusing on keeping your head in a straight line with your back.

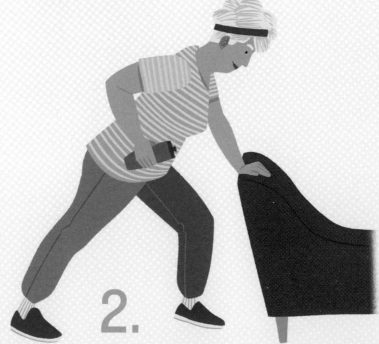

STANDING ROWS

TARGETED MUSCLE GROUPS: Biceps, Latissimus Dorsi, Posterior Deltoid

Do you love to get your hands dirty in the garden? This exercise is the ticket to pain-free gardening. Standing Rows help you lift objects off the floor, start your lawn mower, pull weeds, and push your wheelbarrow and will even make vacuuming easier. Increasing the strength of your arms and upper back also supports your posture and reduces the risk of injuring your shoulders.

INSTRUCTIONS

1. Stand next to a table or chair in a staggered stance with your left leg in front and your right leg behind you. Hold a light weight in your right hand with your elbow extended. Place your left hand on a table or chair for balance and, keeping your back straight, hinge forward from the hips.

2. Keeping your right elbow close to your body, slowly bend your elbow, bringing the weight closer to your chest. Pause at the top of the movement for 1 to 2 seconds, then return to the starting position.

3. Complete 8 to 12 repetitions for 1 set. Do 2 or 3 sets total with 30 to 60 seconds of rest in between sets.

Easy Modification: Use lighter weights and do not hold the contracted position. Instead, momentarily pause, then slowly straighten your elbow, returning to the starting position. In addition, limit how far you bend your elbow until you gain strength.

Challenging Modification: Use heavier weights and hold the contracted position for 3 to 5 seconds before returning to the starting position. To challenge your balance, do the exercise without holding on to a chair for support. You can also do both arms at the same time.

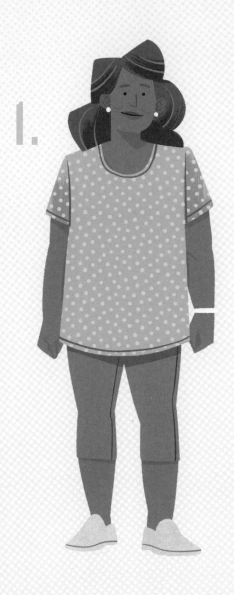

REMEMBER

As you raise your knee toward your chest, stand with a straight back, avoiding the temptation to round your lower back. Stay strong in your support leg, keeping all the muscles tight and contracted and your hips as level as possible.

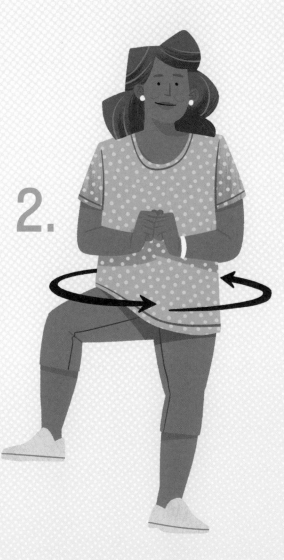

STANDING HIP CIRCLES

TARGETED MUSCLE GROUPS: Glutes, Psoas, Quadriceps

Many of our movements tend to be in a straight line, such as walking and biking, which can lead to hip tightness and pain. Hip circles are a wonderful exercise to improve hip mobility, strength, and balance, and can be used as a warmup or cooldown exercise.

INSTRUCTIONS

1. Stand tall with your core engaged and tighten the muscles of your left leg. Shift your body weight onto your left leg.

2. Clasp your hands together in front of your body. Lift your right knee toward your chest, then rotate your hip outward in a circular motion as far as you can comfortably. Your knee should be bent to about 90 degrees. Then slowly bring your leg back down to the starting position.

3. Complete 8 to 12 repetitions on each hip for 1 set. Do 2 or 3 sets total with 30 to 60 seconds of rest in between sets.

Easy Modification: Use the wall for support or do the hip circles while sitting in a chair. Reducing the range of motion by not lifting your knee as high will also make the exercise easier to do.

Challenging Modification: Place a small weight on your ankle and move more slowly during the exercise. You can also perform more repetitions per set.

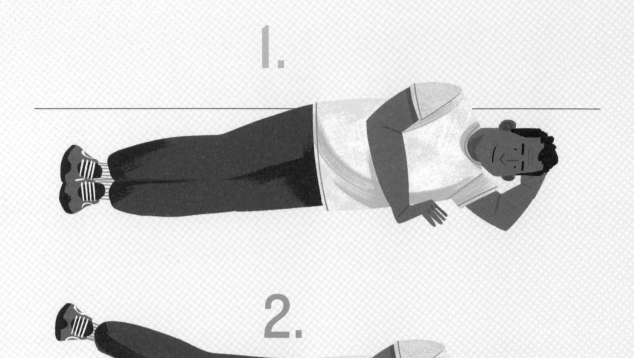

1.

2.

> ### REMEMBER
> Your hips should stay stacked on top of each other throughout the exercise. Keeping your foot parallel to the floor targets the glutes better and helps protect your lower back. The movement should be isolated to the hip by ending the motion when your lower back starts to move.

SIDE-LYING LEG LIFTS

TARGETED MUSCLE GROUP: Glutes

Side-Lying Leg Lifts target the important lateral (outer) hip muscles that are responsible for helping keep your hips level while walking and reducing pain from hip arthritis. Strong lateral hip muscles also improve your side-to-side balance, improving your overall balance and stability.

INSTRUCTIONS

1. Lay on your left side with your head supported by your left arm and your legs in a straight line with your body. Put your right hand on the floor in front of you to help with stabilization.

2. Slowly lift your right leg, keeping your knee locked and your foot parallel to the floor. Pause at the top for 1 to 3 seconds, then return to the starting position.

3. Complete 8 to 12 repetitions on each hip for 1 set. Do 2 or 3 sets per side with 30 to 60 seconds of rest in between sets.

Easy Modification: Reducing the range of motion by not lifting your leg as high will make the exercise easier to do. Remember to keep your foot parallel to the floor.

Challenging Modification: Place a small weight on your ankle and move more slowly during the exercise to increase the time your hip muscles are under tension. You can also perform more repetitions per set.

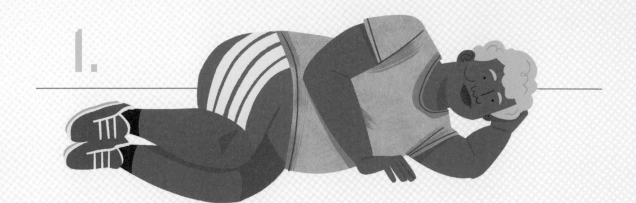

1.

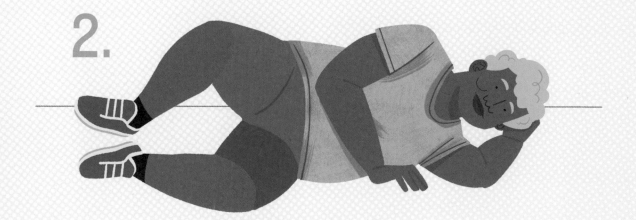

2.

REMEMBER

Engage your core and do not let your pelvis tilt backward during the exercise. Make sure the movement originates from the hips and that there is no rotation at the lower back. You should feel your hip and buttock muscles contracting as you lift your top leg.

CLAMSHELLS

TARGETED MUSCLE GROUP: Glutes

Hip muscle weakness is common as you age. Weakness of the hip can cause poor balance and difficulty walking, increasing your risk of falling. Clamshells are an easy but effective way to strengthen your hips and stabilize your pelvis when walking and climbing stairs.

INSTRUCTIONS

1. Lay on your left side with your head supported by your left arm. Stack your legs on top of each other and bend them slightly. Put your right hand on the floor in front of you to help with stabilization.

2. Keep your feet together and lift your top knee as far as you can comfortably, like the opening of a clam. Pause at the top for 1 to 3 seconds and then return to the starting position.

3. Complete 8 to 12 repetitions on each hip for 1 set. Do 2 or 3 sets per side with 30 to 60 seconds of rest in between sets.

Easy Modification: Reduce the range of motion by not lifting your leg as high. Place a pillow in between your knees, making it easier to lift your top leg.

Challenging Modification: Use a resistance band around your thighs, just above your knees, and move more slowly during the exercise to increase the time under tension of your hip muscles. You can also perform more repetitions per set.

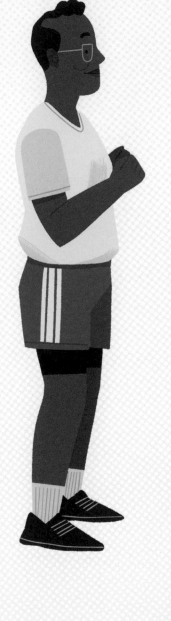

1.

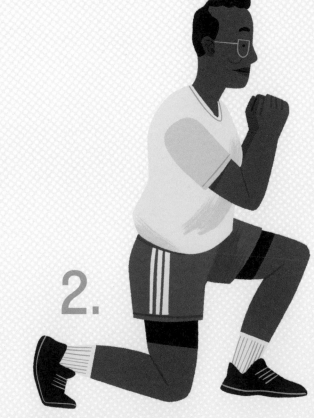

2.

REVERSE LUNGES

TARGETED MUSCLE GROUPS:

Calves, Core Muscles, Glutes, Hamstrings, Quadriceps

Reverse Lunges are a very functional exercise that will improve your balance, core strength, flexibility, and lower-body strength. This will allow you to safely pick up objects from the floor without stressing your lower back.

INSTRUCTIONS

1. Stand with your feet shoulder-width apart, with your core engaged and your hands clasped in front of your body.

2. Keeping your back as straight as you can, take a step backward with your right leg and lower your body until your front knee is bent to about 90 degrees. Your back knee should hover just above the ground. Push through your left heel and return to the starting position.

3. Complete 8 to 12 repetitions on each leg for 1 set. Do 2 or 3 sets per side with 30 to 60 seconds of rest in between sets.

Easy Modification: Decrease the depth of the lunge or hold on to a chair for support. If additional support is needed, you can stand in between two heavy chairs and use both arms for support and balance as needed.

Challenging Modification: Hold small weights in each hand, hold the reverse lunge position for 3 to 5 seconds, or increase the depth of the lunge. You can also increase the number of repetitions or sets.

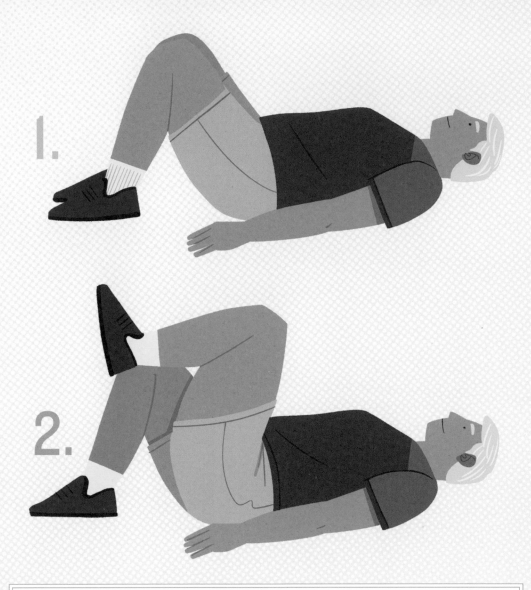

REMEMBER

Keeping your lower back flat on the floor throughout the exercise is essential. As you lift your knee, your lower back will want to arch up. However, keeping your abdominal muscles tight will prevent arching. Exhale as you lift your knee and inhale as you lower it.

SUPINE HEEL RAISES

TARGETED MUSCLE GROUPS: Obliques, Rectus Abdominis

The respiratory diaphragm, our primary breathing muscle, is part of the core, and improved core strength leads to better breathing. Improving core strength also helps maintain good posture, reduces the risk of lower back pain, and helps with daily activities such as getting in and out of bed. It can also improve your reaching abilities, making it easier to grab items from high shelves or low surfaces.

INSTRUCTIONS

1. Lie flat on your back with your knees bent, your feet on the ground, and your arms by your side. Draw your belly button in toward your spine to contract your abdominal muscles and keep your lower back flat on the floor.

2. Slowly lift your left knee toward your chest as far as you can comfortably. Hold this position for 1 to 2 seconds, then return to the starting position. Focus on continuously breathing throughout the exercise rather than holding your breath.

3. Complete 8 to 12 repetitions on each leg for 1 set. Do 2 or 3 sets per side with 30 to 60 seconds of rest in between sets.

Easy Modification: Start by lifting your heels just a few inches off the floor, momentarily pausing, then lower your heel back down. Start with fewer repetitions per set.

Challenging Modification: Place a small weight on each ankle and increase the hold to 3 to 5 seconds. Add additional repetitions to each set.

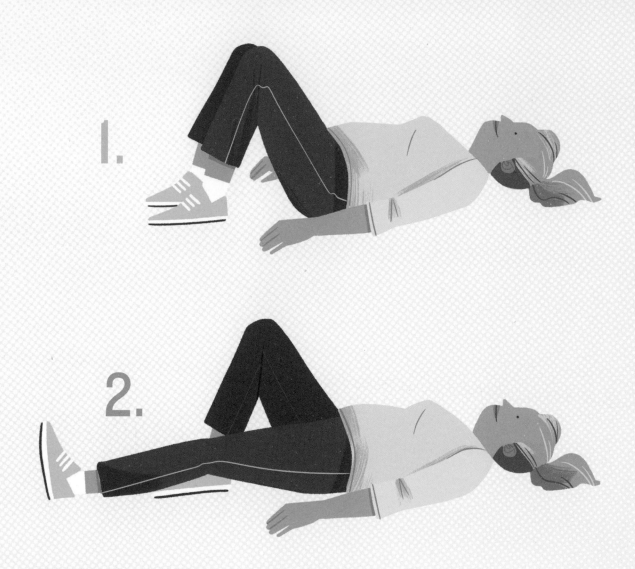

REMEMBER

As you slide your heel down, your lower back will want to arch up. Keep your lower back flat by contracting your abdominals. If your back still begins to arch, stop sliding your heel and return to the starting position. You need to limit your heel slide until your abdominals become stronger.

SUPINE HEEL SLIDES

TARGETED MUSCLE GROUPS: Obliques, Rectus Abdominis

Heel Slides increase the strength and endurance of your core muscles. Improving core strength helps maintain good posture, reduces the risk of lower back pain, improves balance, and helps with daily activities, such as getting up and down from the floor, sweeping the floor, and navigating stairs.

INSTRUCTIONS

1. Lie flat on your back with your knees bent, your feet on the ground, and your arms by your sides. Draw your belly button in toward your spine to contract your abdominal muscles and keep your lower back flat on the floor.

2. Slide your left heel away from your body, straightening your leg while keeping your core muscles contracted and your lower back flat on the floor. Pause for 1 to 2 seconds when your leg is fully extended, then return to the starting position.

3. Complete 8 to 12 repetitions on each leg for 1 set. Do 2 or 3 sets per side with 30 to 60 seconds of rest in between sets.

Easy Modification: Slide your heel a shorter distance from your body, pause, then return to the starting position. Start with a fewer number of repetitions per set.

Challenging Modification: Place a small weight on each ankle or add additional repetitions to each set. You can also allow your foot to hover a few inches off the ground as you slide it away from your body.

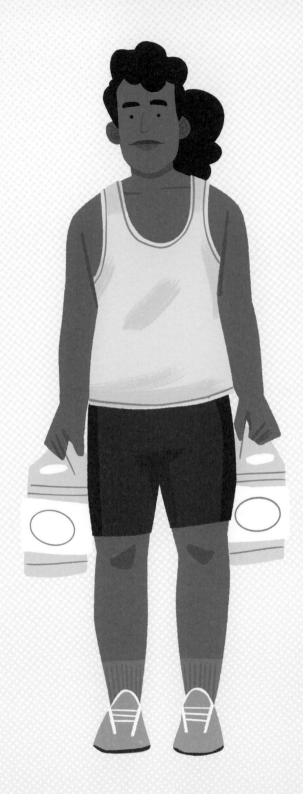

REMEMBER
Use supportive footwear and stand on a nonslip surface. Move smoothly, avoiding any quick or jerky movements, and start with lighter weights. Grip strength may be a limiting factor until your strength improves. Avoid leaning forward and keep the weights close to your body.

FARMER'S WALK

TARGETED MUSCLE GROUPS: Calves, Core Muscles, Glutes, Grip Strength, Hamstrings, Latissimus Dorsi, Spinal Erectors, Trapezius

Farmer's Walk is one of my favorites and can be used as a warm-up exercise. It activates over 200 muscles, engaging multiple muscle groups simultaneously, promoting overall strength and stability, and improving your carrying capacity. By adding weight to each hand and then walking, it mimics real-life activities, such as carrying heavy groceries or luggage or pushing a wheelbarrow.

INSTRUCTIONS

1. Stand tall with your core engaged, with your arms by your side, holding a weight in each hand. Slowly walk forward for a set distance, such as 15 to 20 steps. Turn around, walk back, and put the weights down.

2. Rest for 30 to 60 seconds in between sets and then repeat 2 or 3 times.

Easy Modification: Start with lighter weights in each hand and limit the number of steps you take.

Challenging Modification: Carry heavier weights in your hands and add more steps per set. If you have good balance, you can add stairs to your steps.

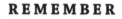

> **REMEMBER**
> Use your leg muscles to lift your body onto the step, rather than pushing off with your toes or using momentum. If you have a harder time going up a step with a particular leg, do a few extra repetitions on the weaker side to improve the strength.

STEP-UPS

TARGETED MUSCLE GROUPS: Calves, Glutes, Hamstrings, Quadriceps

The Step-Up is a very functional leg-strengthening exercise with real-
world implications. Although you may not need to use stairs at your house, maintaining the ability to go up and down steps will keep you strong and independent and allow you to access areas that don't have elevators.

INSTRUCTIONS

1. Stand facing a staircase and, using the railing for balance, step up with your right foot, then your left. Then step down with your right foot, then step down with your left.

2. Repeat 8 to 10 times, leading with your right leg. Then switch and lead with your left foot.

3. Do 2 or 3 sets per leg and rest 30 to 60 seconds in between sets.

Easy Modification: Find a smaller step or reduce the number of repetitions per set. If you don't have steps at home, you may need to seek out a local park or public building that has stairs and a railing. Marching in place is another great alternative.

Challenging Modification: Carry a light weight in your hand or add more steps per set. If you have good balance, you can add a weight to each hand.

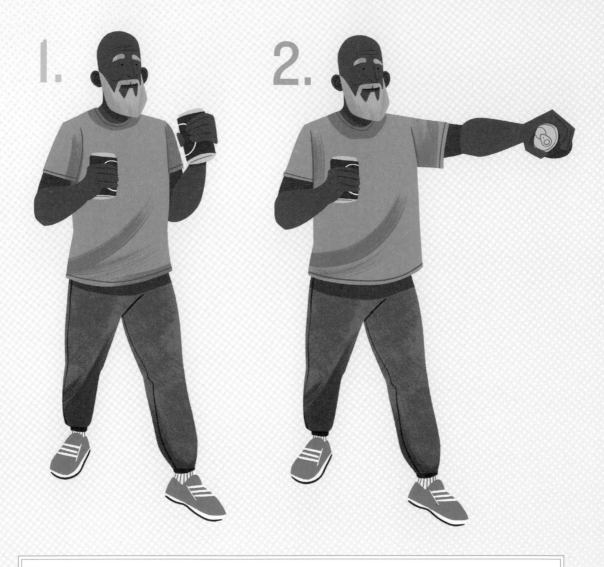

POWER PUNCH

TARGETED MUSCLE GROUPS: Biceps, Core Muscles, Deltoids, Pectoralis, Triceps

A power exercise is one that focuses on generating explosive force and maximizing muscular strength and speed. Power exercises help increase cognitive function, reduce falls by improving your balance and stability, improve muscle mass and strength, and increase cardiorespiratory health. Plus, it's fun to punch!

INSTRUCTIONS

1. Stand in a staggered stance with your left leg forward and right leg back. Holding light weights in each hand, bend your elbows and bring the weights up to your chest.

2. Stand tall and engage your core. Alternate punching with your left and right fists, twisting your torso. Punch at a pace that is quick, but begin with low-intensity punches and gradually increase the intensity over time. This allows the body to adapt and reduces the risk of injury.

3. Complete 8 to 10 punches on each arm, then switch the position of your legs and complete another 8 to 10 repetitions. This constitutes 1 set on each side. Try to repeat for 2 or 3 sets per side with 30 to 60 seconds of rest in between sets.

Easy Modification: Use lighter weights, slow down the pace of the punches, or reduce the number of repetitions per set.

Challenging Modification: Carry a heavier weight in your hand and add more punches per set. Slowly increase the intensity and speed of the punches.

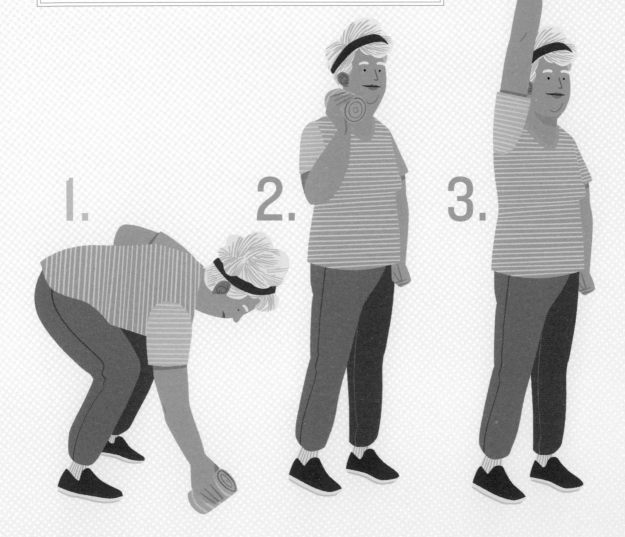

REMEMBER

First do the exercise without weights and without the speed element to become comfortable with the movement. If you experience lower back fatigue or strain, stop the exercise and make sure you are hinging your hips correctly. Use your legs to drive the motion, rather than relying solely on your arms.

I.

2.

3.

SQUAT AND LIFT

TARGETED MUSCLE GROUPS:
Biceps, Core Muscles, Deltoids, Glutes, Pectoralis, Triceps

This multi-joint functional exercise helps strengthen both your upper and lower body at the same time. This is a power exercise, meaning you should perform the movements as quickly as you safely can. Picking up items from the floor and putting them away on a top shelf will become a breeze after doing this exercise.

INSTRUCTIONS

1. Stand with your feet shoulder-width apart and a light weight on the floor in front of you. Hinging at the hips and bending your knees, reach down with one hand and grasp the weight.

2. Stand up quickly, bending your elbow, and bring the weight to your shoulder in one fluid motion.

3. From this position, push the weight overhead until your arm is straight. Pause for 1 to 2 seconds, then bring the weight down to your shoulder, then down to the floor. That is 1 repetition.

4. Complete 6 to 10 repetitions with each arm for 1 set. Do 2 or 3 sets per side and rest for 30 to 60 seconds in between sets.

Easy Modification: Start with the weight on a raised surface so you don't need to reach down to the floor. Use lighter weights, slow down the pace of the movement, or reduce the number of repetitions per set.

Challenging Modification: Use a heavier weight and increase the number of repetitions.

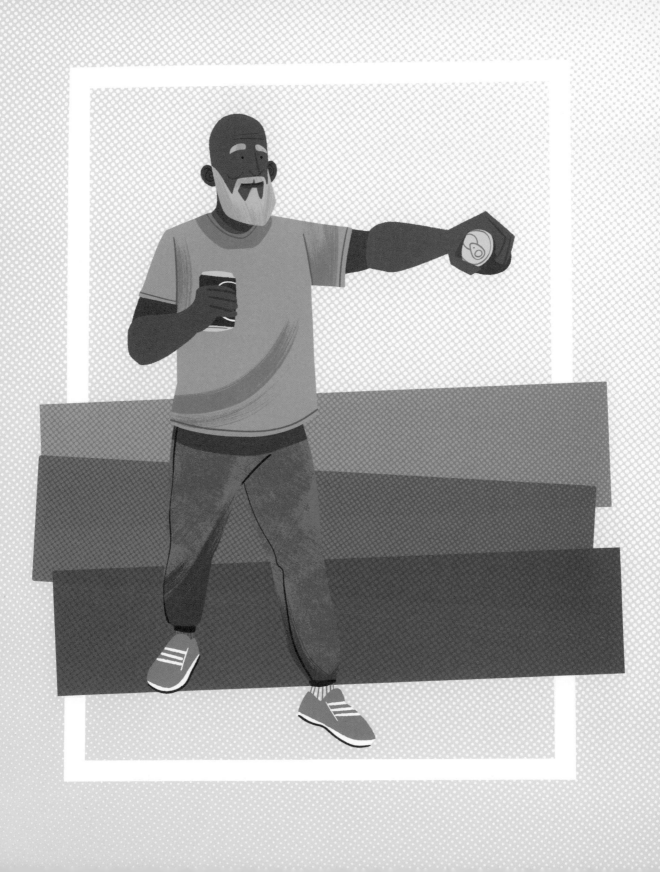

PART THREE

STRENGTH TRAINING
ROUTINES

GET READY TO IGNITE YOUR FITNESS JOURNEY with part 3 of this power-packed book! I provide twenty-five dynamic exercise routines, each designed to invigorate your body and get you stronger in just ten minutes a day. From the strength-building Harvesttime Hustle (page 115) to the high-energy Power Surge (page 125), these routines have you covered from head to toe. Each routine consists of four carefully curated exercises, each explained in part 2, that target specific areas with varying intensity levels.

If you are just starting your fitness journey, or have limited mobility, seated exercises offer a wonderful opportunity to engage in physical activity while seated comfortably. As you progress and your fitness level increases, you can explore intermediate routines that involve standing exercises, incorporating more dynamic movements and increasing the intensity.

But wait, I haven't forgotten about the peak performers! For those craving the ultimate challenge, there are routines that will take your fitness to the next level. Push your limits as you embark on this intense, heart-pounding journey.

Expert guidance ensures safety and optimal results throughout your workout. So, whether you're seated or seeking high-level challenges, you can embark on your journey toward improved health at your own pace. Let's do this!

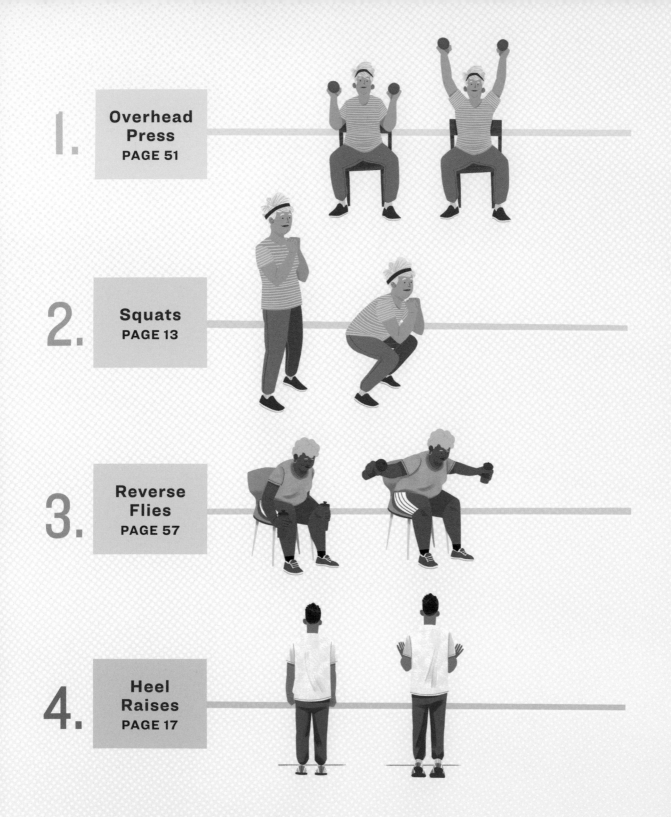

1. Overhead
Press
PAGE 51

2. Squats
PAGE 13

3. Reverse
Flies
PAGE 57

4. Heel
Raises
PAGE 17

TOTAL BODY TUNE-UP

TARGETED BENEFITS:

Endurance, Joint Health, Metabolic Health, Muscle Mass, Posture

Get strong from head to toe by incorporating multi-joint upper- and lower-body exercises. Since these exercises work multiple groups simultaneously, you burn more calories, improve circulation, and improve your metabolic health. Activities such as swimming and tennis require a higher level of physical ability that demands both arm and leg strength. This routine will help you gain strength and endurance in your entire body.

THE ROUTINE

1. **OVERHEAD PRESS:** 8 to 12 repetitions for 2 or 3 sets

   30 to 60 seconds' rest in between sets

2. **SQUATS:** 8 to 12 repetitions for 2 or 3 sets

   30 to 60 seconds' rest in between sets

3. **REVERSE FLIES:** 8 to 12 repetitions for 2 or 3 sets

   30 to 60 seconds' rest in between sets

4. **HEEL RAISES:** 8 to 12 repetitions for 2 or 3 sets

   30 to 60 seconds' rest in between sets

Remember: Alternate between upper- and lower-body exercises to keep your muscles fresh. Keep your core engaged and your back straight during each of the exercises. When squatting, keep your knees aligned with your toes, preventing them from collapsing in.

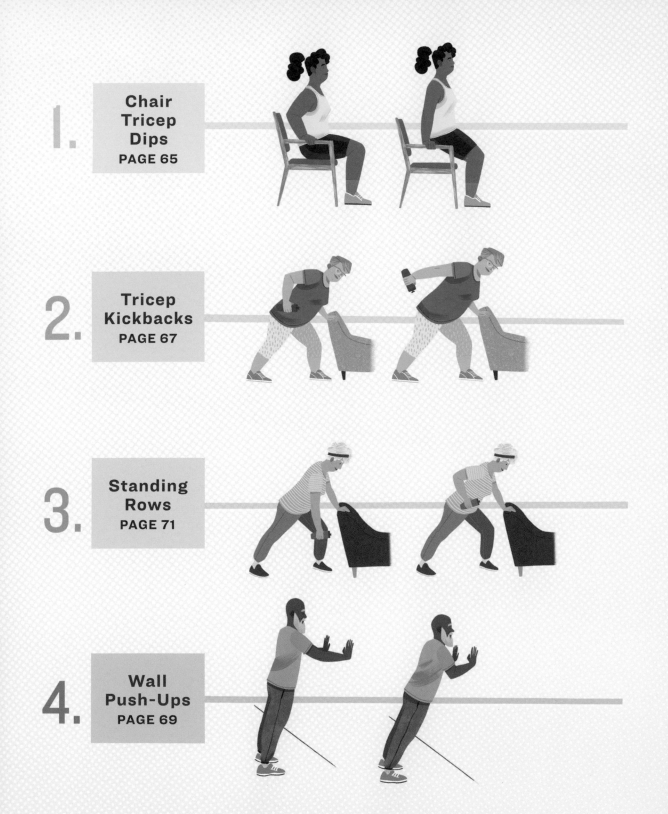

1. Chair Tricep Dips
PAGE 65

2. Tricep Kickbacks
PAGE 67

3. Standing Rows
PAGE 71

4. Wall Push-Ups
PAGE 69

UPPER-BODY BLAST

TARGETED BENEFITS: Bone Density, Joint Health, Mobility, Posture

Power up your arms and chest with this routine, which can have you easily swinging a golf club, swiftly paddleboarding across a serene lake, or effortlessly moving pots and pans around your kitchen. Stronger arms also contribute to better posture, reducing the likelihood of back pain and improving overall alignment. Furthermore, the increased muscle mass boosts your metabolic rate and increases bone density.

THE ROUTINE

1. **CHAIR TRICEP DIPS:** 8 to 12 repetitions for 2 or 3 sets

   30 to 60 seconds' rest in between sets

2. **TRICEP KICKBACKS:** 8 to 12 repetitions for 2 or 3 sets

   30 to 60 seconds' rest in between sets

3. **STANDING ROWS:** 8 to 12 repetitions for 2 or 3 sets

   30 to 60 seconds' rest in between sets

4. **WALL PUSH-UPS:** 8 to 12 repetitions for 2 or 3 sets

   30 to 60 seconds' rest in between sets

Remember: Don't let your lower back round; instead, focus on hinging at the hips and keeping your core engaged. Taking the time to rest in between sets will allow you to give maximum effort during each exercise.

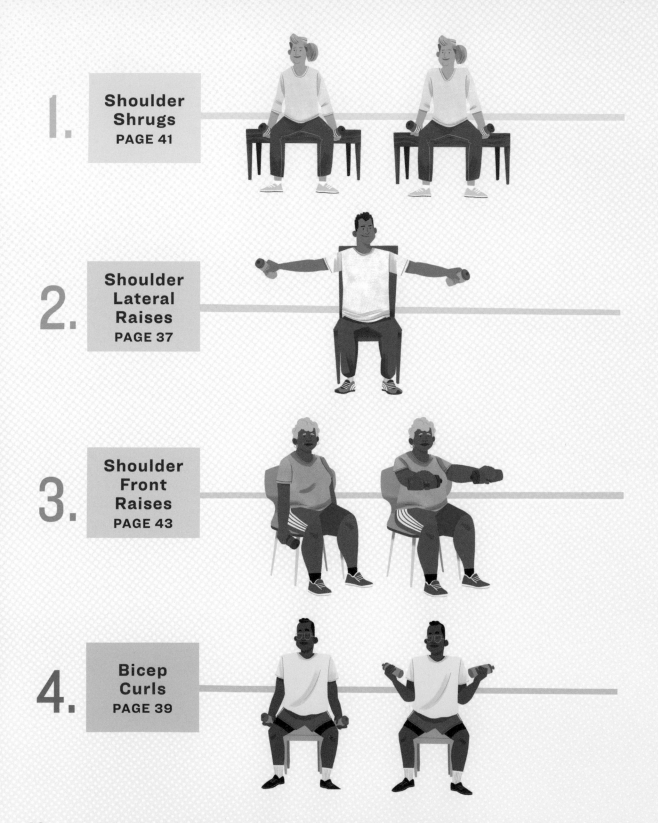

1. Shoulder Shrugs
PAGE 41

2. Shoulder Lateral Raises
PAGE 37

3. Shoulder Front Raises
PAGE 43

4. Bicep Curls
PAGE 39

CHAIR-ROBICS

TARGETED BENEFITS:
Aches and Pains, Endurance, Joint Health, Metabolic Health

Energize your body from the comfort of your favorite chair with this routine designed for those who prefer or require a seated workout. The focus is on upper-body strengthening and endurance to increase blood flow and promote cardiovascular health, boosting energy levels and reducing joint stiffness and pain.

THE ROUTINE

1. **SHOULDER SHRUGS:** 8 to 12 repetitions for 2 or 3 sets

   30 to 60 seconds' rest in between sets

2. **SHOULDER LATERAL RAISES:** 8 to 12 repetitions for 2 or 3 sets

   30 to 60 seconds' rest in between sets

3. **SHOULDER FRONT RAISES:** 8 to 12 repetitions in each direction for 2 or 3 sets

   30 to 60 seconds' rest in between sets

4. **BICEP CURLS:** 8 to 12 repetitions for 2 or 3 sets

   30 to 60 seconds' rest in between sets

Remember: Ensure that your chair is stable and has a supportive backrest. Maintain proper posture with a straight back. Lifting one foot off the ground will help engage your core and help you work on seated balance.

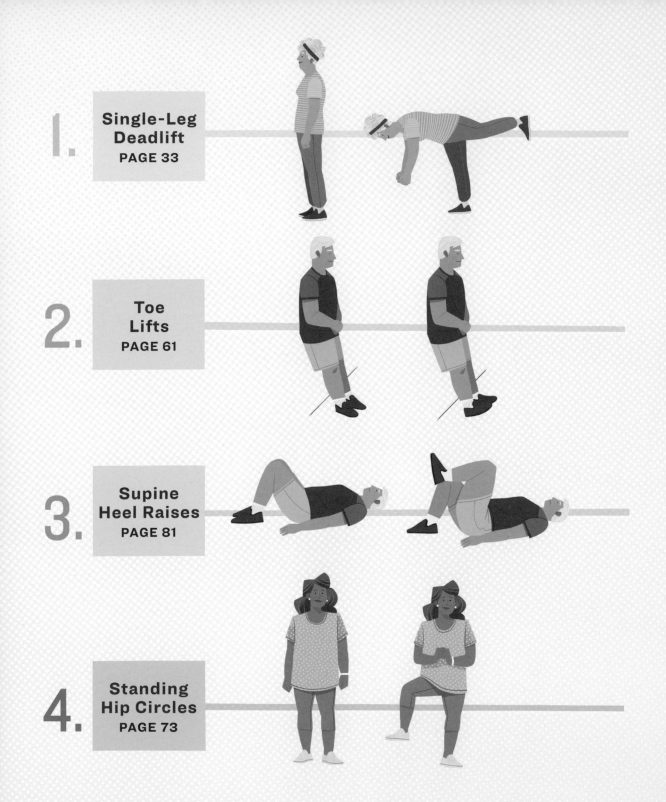

1. Single-Leg Deadlift
PAGE 33

2. Toe Lifts
PAGE 61

3. Supine Heel Raises
PAGE 81

4. Standing Hip Circles
PAGE 73

BALANCE BOOSTER

TARGETED BENEFITS: Balance, Endurance, Mobility

Since the leading cause of hip fractures is falling, working on balance is critical. Step into stability and confidence with this routine, which is all about challenging your balance, improving hip mobility, increasing ankle strength, and enhancing proprioception, or your body awareness in space. It allows you to know how your body is moving, even without looking.

THE ROUTINE

1. **SINGLE-LEG DEADLIFT:** 8 to 12 repetitions for 2 or 3 sets

   30 to 60 seconds' rest in between sets

2. **TOE LIFTS:** 8 to 12 repetitions for 2 or 3 sets

   30 to 60 seconds' rest in between sets

3. **SUPINE HEEL RAISES:** 8 to 12 repetitions for 2 or 3 sets

   30 to 60 seconds' rest in between sets

4. **STANDING HIP CIRCLES:** 8 to 12 repetitions for 2 or 3 sets

   30 to 60 seconds' rest in between sets

Remember: Since we are focusing on challenging our sense of balance with these exercises, use the least amount of support needed. During the Single-Leg Deadlift, keep your back straight by hinging your hips, and do not round your lower back.

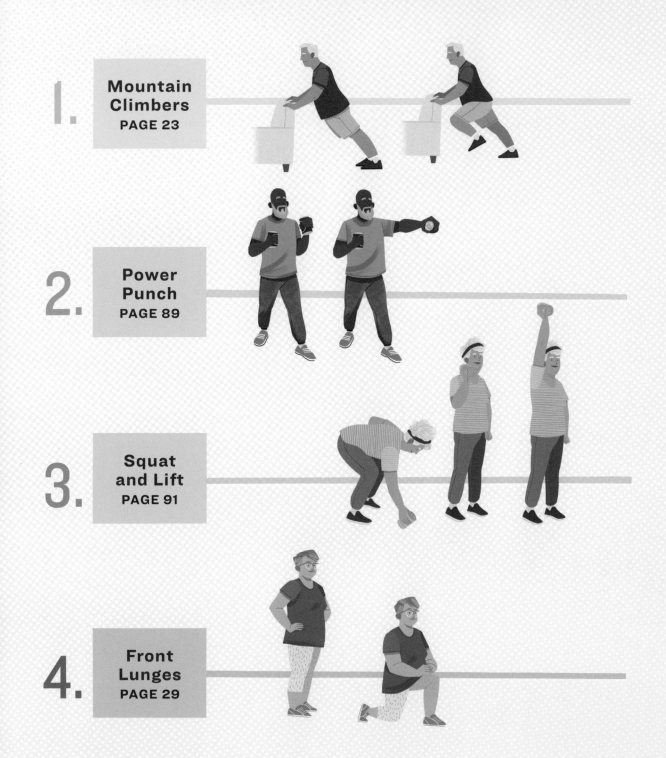

I. Mountain Climbers
PAGE 23

2. Power Punch
PAGE 89

3. Squat and Lift
PAGE 91

4. Front Lunges
PAGE 29

CARDIO KICK START

TARGETED BENEFITS: Balance, Bone Density, Endurance, Metabolic Health

Get your heart pumping, boost your metabolism, and energize your entire body with this routine focusing on high-intensity movements that engage multiple muscle groups. It provides a great cardio workout, leading to improved metabolic health. Practicing moving your arms and feet quickly helps enhance reaction time, an essential component of improving balance and helping your tennis game!

THE ROUTINE

1. **MOUNTAIN CLIMBERS:** 8 to 12 repetitions for 2 or 3 sets

    30 to 60 seconds' rest in between sets

2. **POWER PUNCH:** 8 to 10 repetitions for 2 or 3 sets

    30 to 60 seconds' rest in between sets

3. **SQUAT AND LIFT:** 6 to 10 repetitions for 2 or 3 sets

    30 to 60 seconds' rest in between sets

4. **FRONT LUNGES:** 8 to 10 repetitions for 2 or 3 sets

    30 to 60 seconds' rest in between sets

Remember: Focus on maintaining proper form and intensity throughout the routine. Start at a comfortable pace and gradually increase the speed and intensity as your fitness level improves. The goal is to move as fast as you can safely.

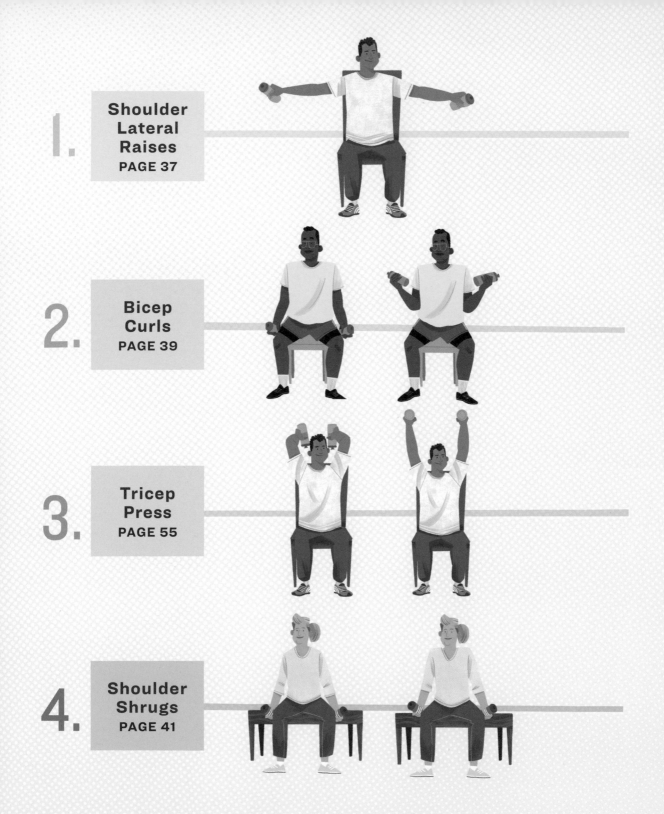

1. Shoulder Lateral Raises PAGE 37

2. Bicep Curls PAGE 39

3. Tricep Press PAGE 55

4. Shoulder Shrugs PAGE 41

ARM ATTACK

TARGETED BENEFITS: Aches and Pains, Joint Health, Mobility, Muscle Mass

Unleash the power of your upper body with this routine that is all about shoulder health, improving your mobility, and reducing pain. Activities such as reaching overhead, carrying luggage, and playing sports heavily rely on the strength and mobility of our shoulders. Age-related decline in arm strength can make your shoulders more vulnerable to injury. The muscles in your arms, particularly the biceps and triceps, play a critical role in stabilizing the shoulder joint during movement. This routine will ensure that your shoulders remain healthy and pain-free.

THE ROUTINE

1. **SHOULDER LATERAL RAISES:** 8 to 12 repetitions for 2 or 3 sets

   30 to 60 seconds' rest in between sets

2. **BICEP CURLS:** 8 to 12 repetitions for 2 or 3 sets

   30 to 60 seconds' rest in between sets

3. **TRICEP PRESS:** 8 to 12 repetitions for 2 or 3 sets

   30 to 60 seconds' rest in between sets

4. **SHOULDER SHRUGS:** 8 to 12 repetitions for 2 or 3 sets

   30 to 60 seconds' rest in between sets

Remember: Use slow and controlled movements throughout the range of motion. Focus on keeping your shoulder blades back and down and your core engaged.

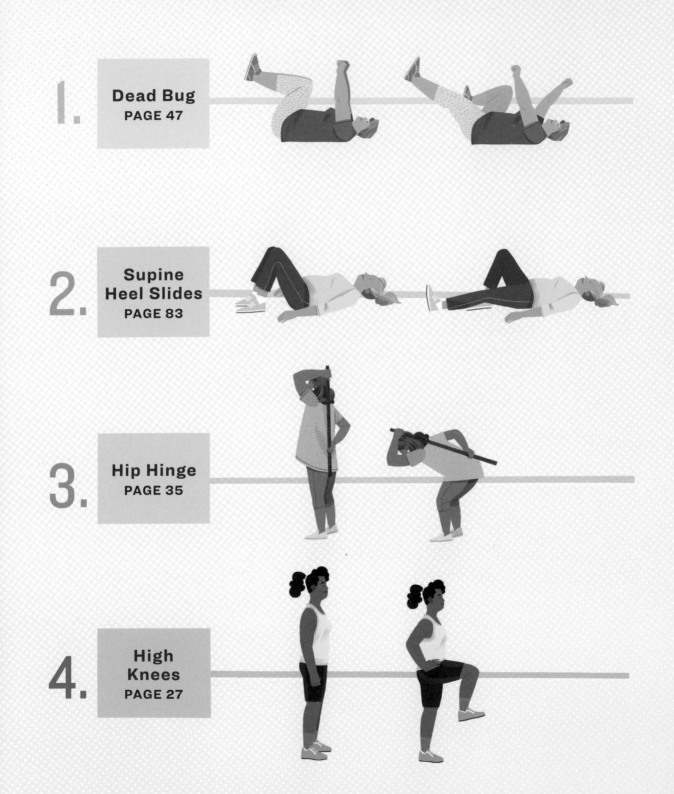

1. Dead Bug
PAGE 47

2. Supine
Heel Slides
PAGE 83

3. Hip Hinge
PAGE 35

4. High
Knees
PAGE 27

CORE CRUSHER

TARGETED BENEFITS: Aches and Pains, Balance, Bone Density, Endurance

You can help improve the bone density in your spine by engaging core muscles, which indirectly stimulates bone growth and promotes overall bone health. In addition, a strong core enhances balance by providing a stable foundation. Build bone density, reduce lower back pain, and improve your balance with this routine. Enhanced core strength and stability leads to improved posture, reducing strain on your spine and alleviating lower back pain.

THE ROUTINE

1. **DEAD BUG:** 8 to 10 repetitions for 2 or 3 sets

   30 to 60 seconds' rest in between sets

2. **SUPINE HEEL SLIDES:** 8 to 12 repetitions for 2 or 3 sets

   30 to 60 seconds' rest in between sets

3. **HIP HINGE:** 8 to 12 repetitions for 2 or 3 sets

   30 to 60 seconds' rest in between sets

4. **HIGH KNEES:** 8 to 12 repetitions for 2 or 3 sets

   30 to 60 seconds' rest in between sets

Remember: Maintain a steady breathing pattern and keep your focus on tightening your abdominal muscles. If you are new to core training, start with shorter durations or easier versions and gradually increase the intensity as you get stronger.

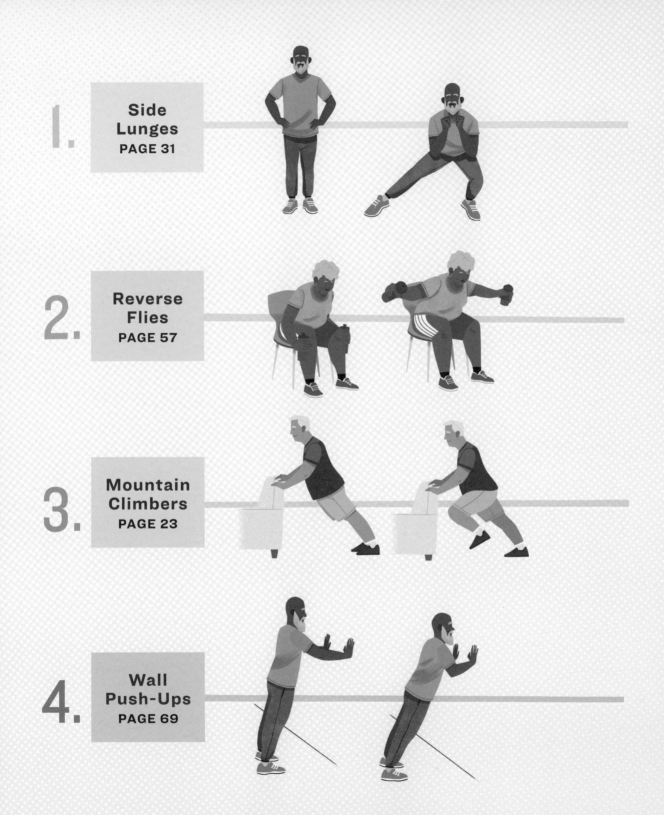

1. Side
Lunges
PAGE 31

2. Reverse
Flies
PAGE 57

3. Mountain
Climbers
PAGE 23

4. Wall
Push-Ups
PAGE 69

COURT CRUSHER

TARGETED BENEFITS: Bone Density, Metabolic Health

Are you one of the millions of people who love racquet sports? Then this dynamic routine designed to target the essentials for dominating the court is for you! Mountain Climbers will enhance your foot quickness and hip strength for improved lateral movement, and the upper-body strengthening will take your smashes to the next level.

THE ROUTINE

1. **SIDE LUNGES:** 8 to 12 repetitions for 2 or 3 sets

   30 to 60 seconds' rest in between sets

2. **REVERSE FLIES:** 8 to 12 repetitions for 2 or 3 sets

   30 to 60 seconds' rest in between sets

3. **MOUNTAIN CLIMBERS:** 8 to 12 repetitions for 2 or 3 sets

   30 to 60 seconds' rest in between sets

4. **WALL PUSH-UPS:** 8 to 12 repetitions for 2 or 3 sets

   30 to 60 seconds' rest in between sets

Remember: Alternating between upper- and lower-body exercises will keep your muscles fresh, and it will allow you to maximize effort. Since these exercises are all about power, as you get comfortable with the routine, increase your speed to as fast as you can safely, prioritizing quick feet and arm movements.

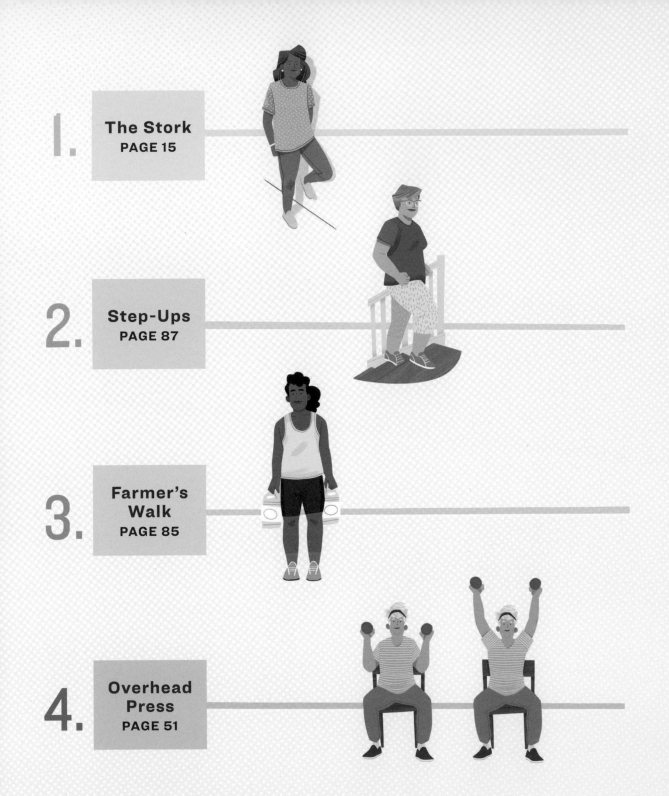

1. **The Stork**
PAGE 15

2. **Step-Ups**
PAGE 87

3. **Farmer's Walk**
PAGE 85

4. **Overhead Press**
PAGE 51

BONE BOOSTER

TARGETED BENEFITS: Balance, Bone Density, Metabolic Health

It is normal to lose bone density as you age, but you can help improve your bone health with strength training and weight-bearing exercises. Build strong bones and become unbreakable with this routine focusing on building the muscles involved with walking, strengthening your hips for better side-to-side mobility, improving power to help you climb stairs, and enhancing balance.

THE ROUTINE

1. **THE STORK:** Hold for 10 to 15 seconds per set for 2 or 3 sets on each side

   30 to 60 seconds' rest in between sets

2. **STEP-UPS:** 8 to 10 repetitions for 2 or 3 sets

   30 to 60 seconds' rest in between sets

3. **FARMER'S WALK:** 15 to 20 steps per set for 2 or 3 sets

   30 to 60 seconds' rest in between sets

4. **OVERHEAD PRESS:** 8 to 12 repetitions for 2 or 3 sets

   30 to 60 seconds' rest in between sets

Remember: The Stork is a great warm-up and can be done first, getting you ready for the more challenging Farmer's Walk and Step-Ups. Keep the weights in each hand equal when doing the Farmer's Walk, and remember to add weight to challenge yourself as you get stronger.

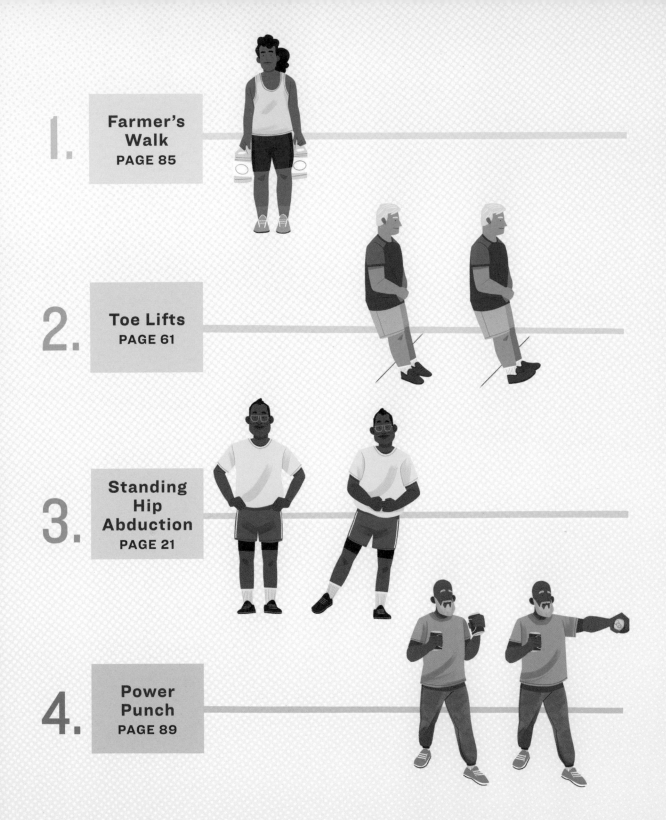

1. **Farmer's Walk**
PAGE 85

2. **Toe Lifts**
PAGE 61

3. **Standing Hip Abduction**
PAGE 21

4. **Power Punch**
PAGE 89

WALKING STRONG

TARGETED BENEFITS: Balance, Endurance, Metabolic Health

Walking daily for 20 to 30 minutes is great for long-term health because it improves cardiovascular and metabolic health and helps maintain strong bones. However, difficulty walking often occurs because of lower-body weakness and ankle stiffness. This routine consists of exercises that improve reaction times for balance and safety, increase ankle strength to prevent shuffling, and develop power in your hips to propel you up hills and stairs. Stride with confidence and stability after this routine.

THE ROUTINE

1. **FARMER'S WALK:** 15 to 20 steps per set for 2 or 3 sets

    30 to 60 seconds' rest in between sets

2. **TOE LIFTS:** 8 to 12 repetitions for 2 or 3 sets on each side

    30 to 60 seconds' rest in between sets

3. **STANDING HIP ABDUCTION:** 8 to 10 repetitions for 2 or 3 sets

    30 to 60 seconds' rest in between sets

4. **POWER PUNCH:** 8 to 10 repetitions for 2 or 3 sets

    30 to 60 seconds' rest in between sets

Remember: Incorporate these exercises into your warm-up routine before you go for a walk, and gradually increase the duration and intensity as your strength and endurance improve. When you become more comfortable with the Power Punch, increase the speed and force of your punches.

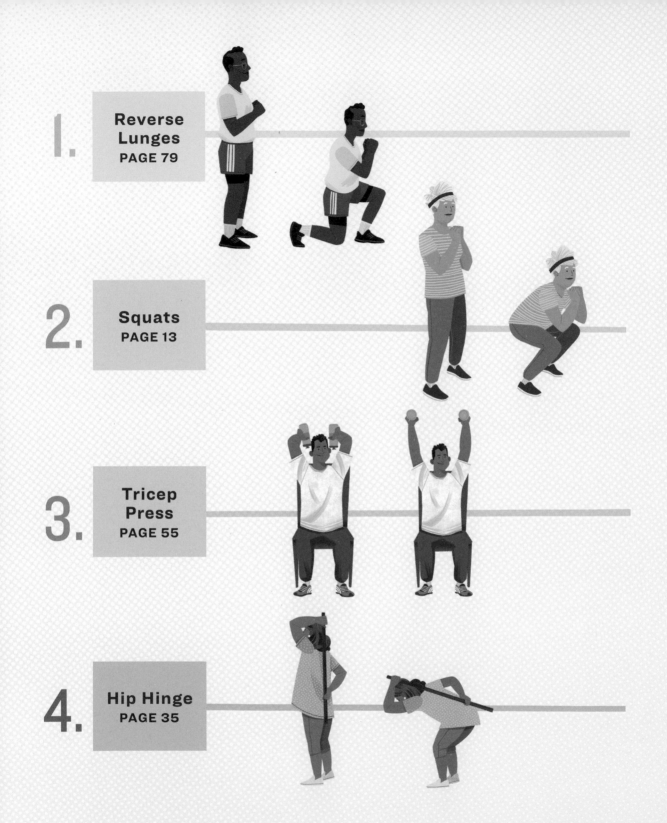

1. Reverse Lunges
PAGE 79

2. Squats
PAGE 13

3. Tricep Press
PAGE 55

4. Hip Hinge
PAGE 35

HARVESTTIME HUSTLE

TARGETED BENEFITS: Aches and Pains, Endurance, Mobility

Gardening gets you outside digging in the dirt, helping you feel better and reducing stress. This routine is designed to prepare your body for the physical demands of working in the garden, reducing your risk of back and hip pain. By focusing on squats, lunges, and safe bending techniques, you'll develop the strength, flexibility, and endurance necessary to garden like a pro.

THE ROUTINE

1. **REVERSE LUNGES:** 8 to 12 repetitions for 2 or 3 sets

   30 to 60 seconds' rest in between sets

2. **SQUATS:** 8 to 12 repetitions for 2 or 3 sets

   30 to 60 seconds' rest in between sets

3. **TRICEP PRESS:** 8 to 12 repetitions for 2 or 3 sets

   30 to 60 seconds' rest in between sets

4. **HIP HINGE:** 8 to 12 repetitions for 2 or 3 sets

   30 to 60 seconds' rest in between sets

Remember: These exercises are best done with a slow and controlled pattern and your core engaged. Prioritize stability during the squats by keeping your feet grounded and chest lifted.

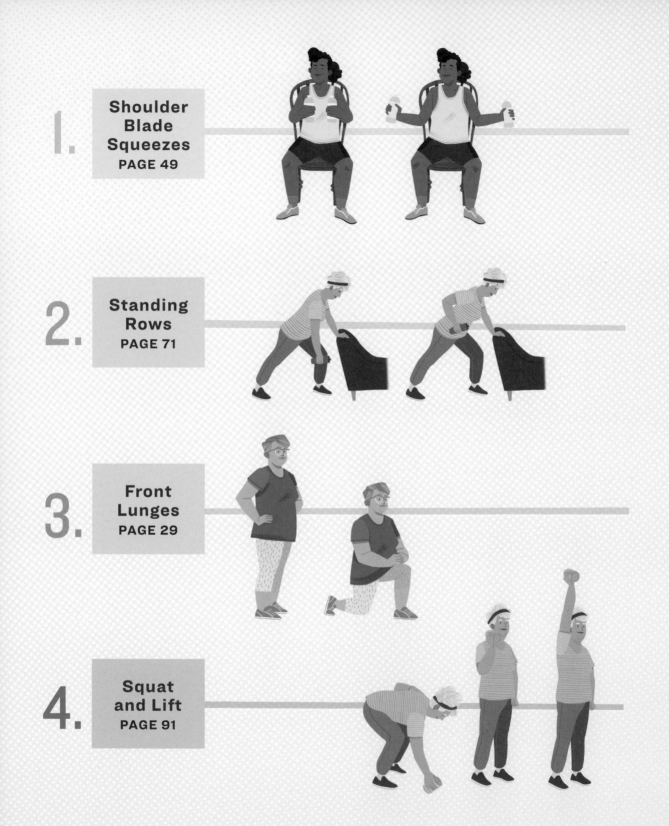

1. Shoulder Blade Squeezes
PAGE 49

2. Standing Rows
PAGE 71

3. Front Lunges
PAGE 29

4. Squat and Lift
PAGE 91

THE MIGHTY MOVER

TARGETED BENEFITS: Bone Density, Endurance, Mobility, Posture

Pushing a wheelbarrow through your yard, doing some spring cleaning, or moving boxes in your garage will become a breeze with this routine by focusing on both upper- and lower-body strength and endurance. Develop the strong hips, back, and core needed to keep you safe and injury free, capable of tackling any project.

THE ROUTINE

1. **SHOULDER BLADE SQUEEZES:** 8 to 12 repetitions for 2 or 3 sets

   30 to 60 seconds' rest in between sets

2. **STANDING ROWS:** 8 to 12 repetitions for 2 or 3 sets

   30 to 60 seconds' rest in between sets

3. **FRONT LUNGES:** 8 to 12 repetitions for 2 or 3 sets

   30 to 60 seconds' rest in between sets

4. **SQUAT AND LIFT:** 6 to 10 repetitions for 2 or 3 sets

   30 to 60 seconds' rest in between sets

Remember: Keep your spine straight, core engaged, and hinge at the hips. Execute the Squat and Lift exercise slowly at first, then gradually increase your speed when you feel comfortable with the movement and your strength improves.

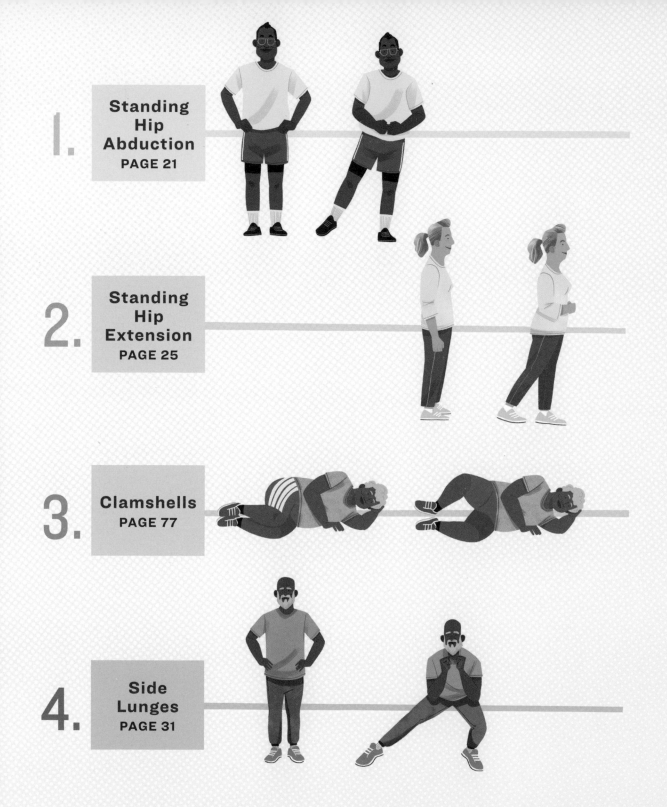

1. Standing Hip Abduction **PAGE 21**

2. Standing Hip Extension **PAGE 25**

3. Clamshells **PAGE 77**

4. Side Lunges **PAGE 31**

HIP HIP HOORAY

TARGETED BENEFITS: Aches and Pains, Balance, Joint Health

Say goodbye to achy, painful hips with this routine designed to reduce hip pain, increase strength, and make daily tasks, such as squatting, walking, and climbing stairs, easier by focusing on hip strength and core stability. Strengthening hip muscles also promotes joint health and contributes to better balance and stability, reducing the risk of falls and injury.

THE ROUTINE

1. **STANDING HIP ABDUCTION:** 8 to 12 repetitions for 2 or 3 sets

   30 to 60 seconds' rest in between sets

2. **STANDING HIP EXTENSION:** 8 to 12 repetitions for 2 or 3 sets

   30 to 60 seconds' rest in between sets

3. **CLAMSHELLS:** 8 to 12 repetitions for 2 or 3 sets

   30 to 60 seconds' rest in between sets

4. **SIDE LUNGES:** 8 to 12 repetitions for 2 or 3 sets

   30 to 60 seconds' rest in between sets

Remember: With the Standing Hip Abduction and Extension exercises, keep your hips level, making sure the movement is originating from the hips, and stop when you feel your lower back starting to get involved.

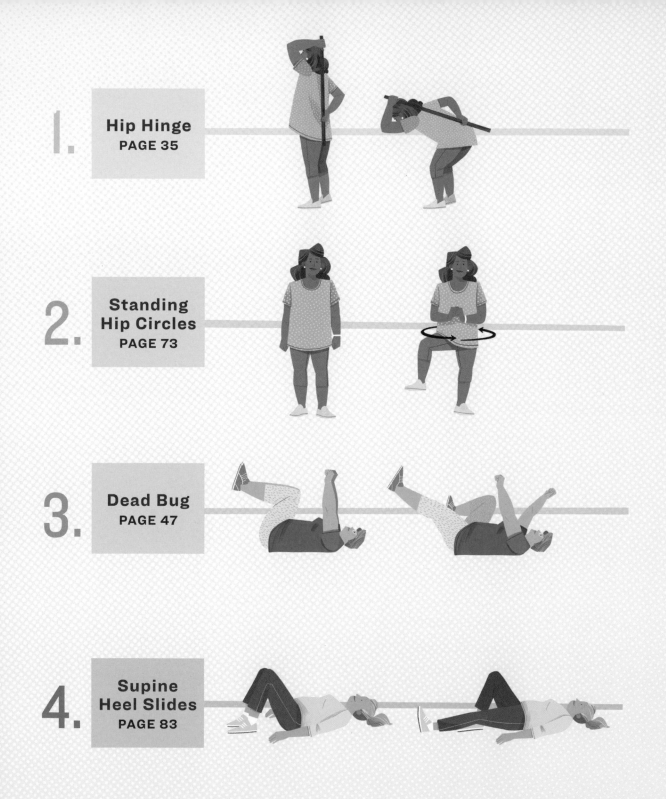

1. Hip Hinge
PAGE 35

2. Standing
Hip Circles
PAGE 73

3. Dead Bug
PAGE 47

4. Supine
Heel Slides
PAGE 83

BACK IN ACTION

TARGETED BENEFITS: Aches and Pains, Balance, Mobility

Nothing stops you in your tracks and dampens your spirits like lower back pain. This routine addresses multiple aspects of back health, including core strength, proper movement patterns, and improved hip mobility to make back pain a thing of the past.

THE ROUTINE

1. **HIP HINGE:** 8 to 12 repetitions for 2 or 3 sets

   30 to 60 seconds' rest in between sets

2. **STANDING HIP CIRCLES:** 8 to 12 repetitions for 2 or 3 sets

   30 to 60 seconds' rest in between sets

3. **DEAD BUG:** 8 to 10 repetitions for 2 or 3 sets

   30 to 60 seconds' rest in between sets

4. **SUPINE HEEL SLIDES:** 8 to 12 repetitions for 2 or 3 sets

   30 to 60 seconds' rest in between sets

Remember: Try to use the Hip Hinge in your daily life every time you need to bend forward. During the Dead Bug and Supine Heel Slides, make sure your lower back stays in contact with the floor. Stop the exercise or make it easier if you feel your lower back arching.

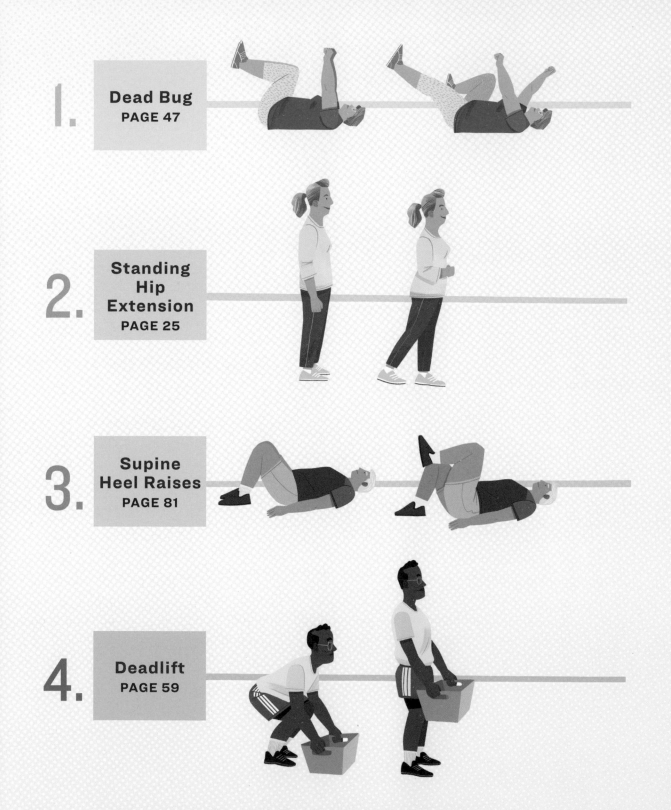

1. **Dead Bug**
PAGE 47

2. **Standing Hip Extension**
PAGE 25

3. **Supine Heel Raises**
PAGE 81

4. **Deadlift**
PAGE 59

STRONG BACK-SAFE LIFTS

TARGETED BENEFITS: Aches and Pains, Bone Density, Endurance, Muscle Mass

If you've ever experienced the agony of injuring your back when lifting something off the floor, you are not alone. Improper lifting techniques and weak core muscles are common culprits behind these painful episodes. This routine aims to empower you with the knowledge and exercises necessary to protect your back and build a resilient core. By increasing core strength and learning to lift correctly, you can reduce the risk of injury, alleviate lower back pain, and gain confidence in daily tasks.

THE ROUTINE

1. **DEAD BUG:** 8 to 10 repetitions for 2 or 3 sets

   30 to 60 seconds' rest in between sets

2. **STANDING HIP EXTENSION:** 8 to 12 repetitions for 2 or 3 sets

   30 to 60 seconds' rest in between sets

3. **SUPINE HEEL RAISES:** 8 to 12 repetitions for 2 or 3 sets

   30 to 60 seconds' rest in between sets

4. **DEADLIFT:** 8 to 12 repetitions for 2 or 3 sets

   30 to 60 seconds' rest in between sets

Remember: During the Deadlift, imagine you are pushing feet into the ground, rather than lifting with your arms. This will take further stress off your back and help you gain strength in your hips and lower back.

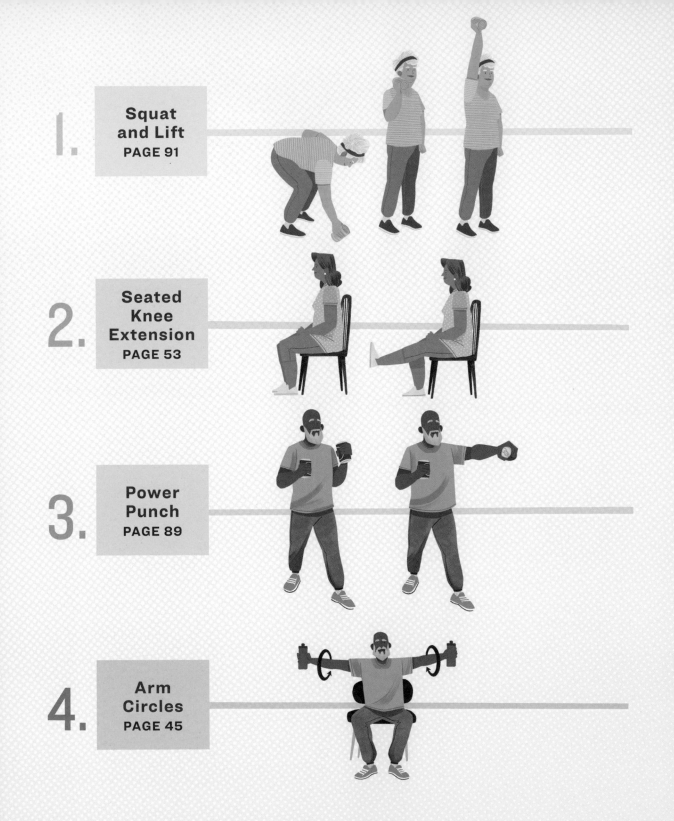

1. **Squat and Lift**
   PAGE 91

2. **Seated Knee Extension**
   PAGE 53

3. **Power Punch**
   PAGE 89

4. **Arm Circles**
   PAGE 45

POWER SURGE

TARGETED BENEFITS: Balance, Endurance, Metabolic Health

Feeling a bit low energy? This high-energy routine is designed to revitalize your energy levels, boost your power, increase your muscular endurance, and sharpen your reaction times for better balance. Using a combination of upper- and lower-body exercises that emphasize power, safe lifting technique, and muscular endurance, you'll be ready for any challenge!

THE ROUTINE

1. **SQUAT AND LIFT:** 6 to 10 repetitions for 2 or 3 sets

   30 to 60 seconds' rest in between sets

2. **SEATED KNEE EXTENSION:** 8 to 12 repetitions for 2 or 3 sets

   30 to 60 seconds' rest in between sets

3. **POWER PUNCH:** 8 to 10 repetitions for 2 or 3 sets

   30 to 60 seconds' rest in between sets

4. **ARM CIRCLES:** 8 to 12 repetitions for 2 or 3 sets

   30 to 60 seconds' rest in between sets

Remember: This routine is all about power and moving as fast as you can safely. When you feel comfortable with the exercises, increase the intensity and the speed of the movements.

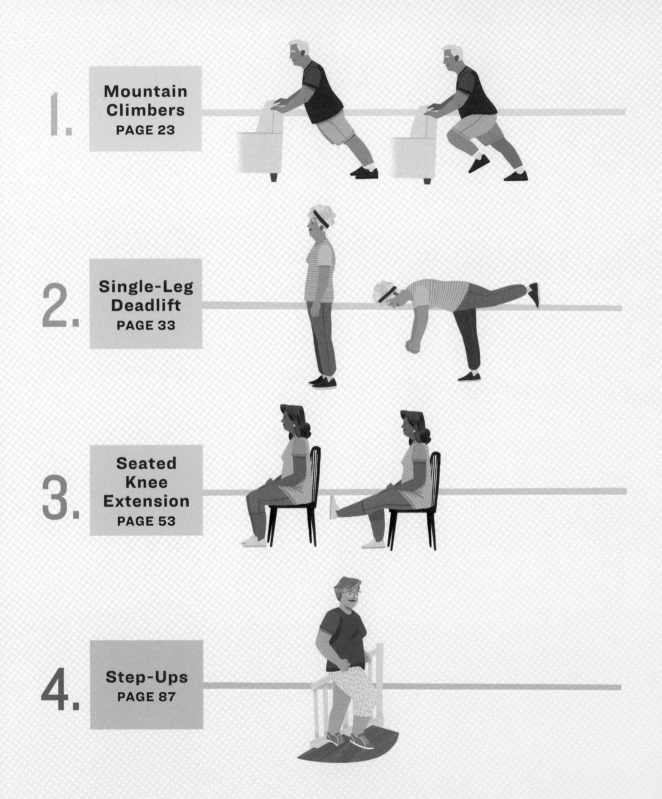

1. **Mountain Climbers** PAGE 23

2. **Single-Leg Deadlift** PAGE 33

3. **Seated Knee Extension** PAGE 53

4. **Step-Ups** PAGE 87

THE TRAILBLAZER

TARGETED BENEFITS: Endurance, Energy, Mobility

Designed for those who love to be outside camping, biking, and hiking, this routine will not only help you stay fit but also elevate your sense of adventure, stimulate your immune system, improve your mental health, and allow you to continue exploring the world around you. By combining exercises that work on balance, power, strength, and reaction times, you will build the confidence to conquer any outdoor adventure.

THE ROUTINE

1. **MOUNTAIN CLIMBERS:** 8 to 12 repetitions for 2 or 3 sets

   30 to 60 seconds' rest in between sets

2. **SINGLE-LEG DEADLIFT:** 8 to 12 repetitions for 2 or 3 sets on each leg

   30 to 60 seconds' rest in between sets

3. **SEATED KNEE EXTENSION:** 8 to 12 repetitions for 2 or 3 sets

   30 to 60 seconds' rest in between sets

4. **STEP-UPS:** 8 to 12 repetitions for 2 or 3 sets

   30 to 60 seconds' rest in between sets

Remember: Since we are working on increasing speed with the Mountain Climbers and Step-Ups, increase your pace as you become comfortable and really challenge yourself. Remember to wear supportive footwear with good traction.

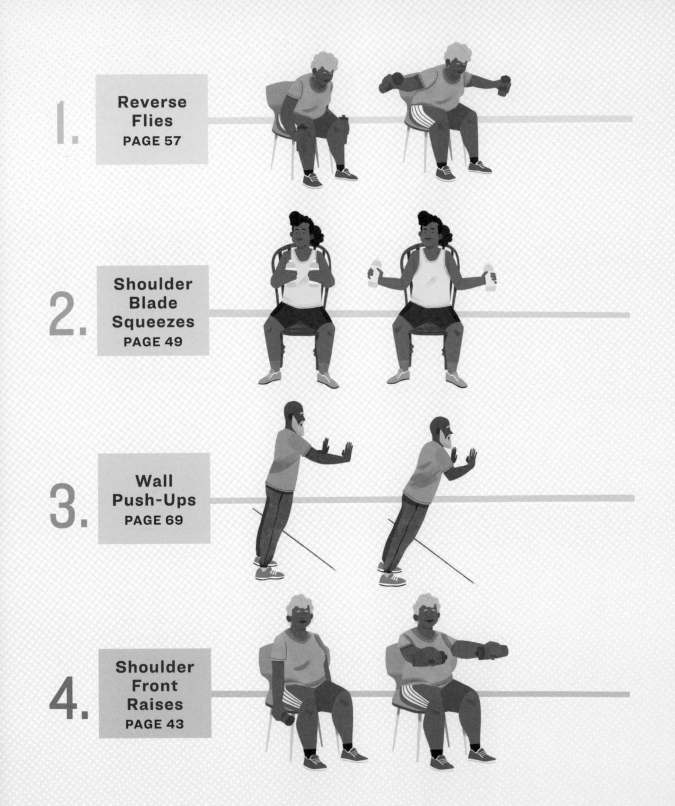

1. Reverse Flies
PAGE 57

2. Shoulder Blade Squeezes
PAGE 49

3. Wall Push-Ups
PAGE 69

4. Shoulder Front Raises
PAGE 43

PERFECT POSTURE

TARGETED BENEFITS: Aches and Pains, Endurance, Mobility

Look and feel better with this routine aimed at perfecting your posture. Improving posture can positively impact mental health by promoting self-confidence and enhancing overall mood and well-being. Poor posture is often caused by weak upper back muscles. This routine targets upper-body strength, specifically the muscles surrounding the shoulder blades, promoting improved posture and reducing the risk of shoulder and neck pain.

THE ROUTINE

1. **REVERSE FLIES:** 8 to 12 repetitions for 2 or 3 sets

   30 to 60 seconds' rest in between sets

2. **SHOULDER BLADE SQUEEZES:** 8 to 12 repetitions for 2 or 3 sets

   30 to 60 seconds' rest in between sets

3. **WALL PUSH-UPS:** 8 to 12 repetitions for 2 or 3 sets

   30 to 60 seconds' rest in between sets

4. **SHOULDER FRONT RAISES:** 8 to 12 repetitions for 2 or 3 sets

   30 to 60 seconds' rest in between sets

Remember: Keep your shoulder blades back and down during all the exercises, and feel the muscles in between your shoulder blades contract. Your neck is straight, aligned with your back, and you are not looking up or down.

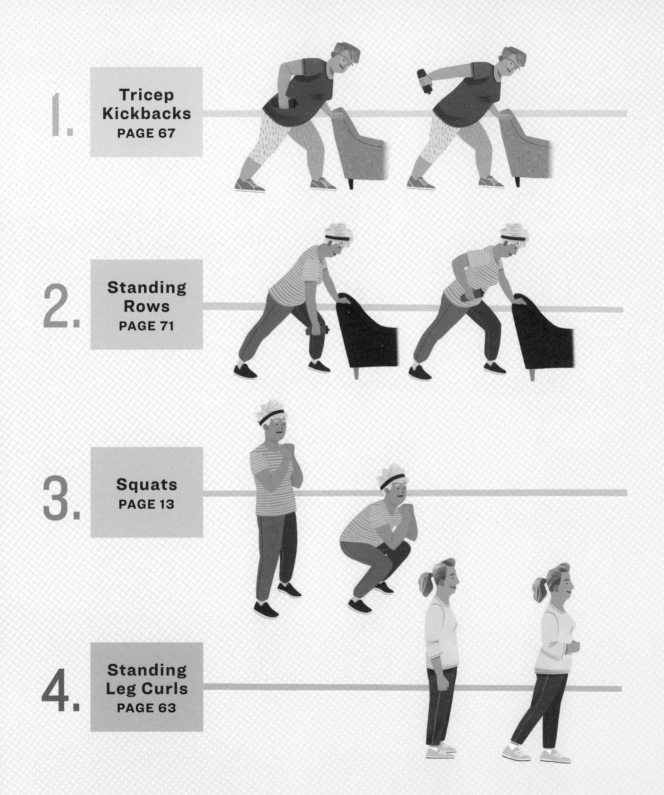

1. Tricep
Kickbacks
PAGE 67

2. Standing
Rows
PAGE 71

3. Squats
PAGE 13

4. Standing
Leg Curls
PAGE 63

ROAD WARRIOR

TARGETED BENEFITS: Balance, Mobility

Ready for adventure? Conquer the road and unleash your strength with this routine. Being on the road requires the ability to have both upper- and lower-body strength to lift, pack, and climb. This routine combines exercises to improve your upper body's pulling and pushing muscles, develop power in your legs, and enhance your single-leg balance for fall prevention.

THE ROUTINE

1. **TRICEP KICKBACKS:** 8 to 12 repetitions for 2 or 3 sets

   30 to 60 seconds' rest in between sets

2. **STANDING ROWS:** 8 to 12 repetitions for 2 or 3 sets

   30 to 60 seconds' rest in between sets

3. **SQUATS:** 8 to 12 repetitions for 2 or 3 sets

   30 to 60 seconds' rest in between sets

4. **STANDING LEG CURLS:** 8 to 12 repetitions for 2 or 3 sets

   30 to 60 seconds' rest in between sets

Remember: If you feel any strain in your lower back, stop the exercise and make sure you are correctly hinging at the hips. Gradually increase the weights as you become stronger to keep gaining strength!

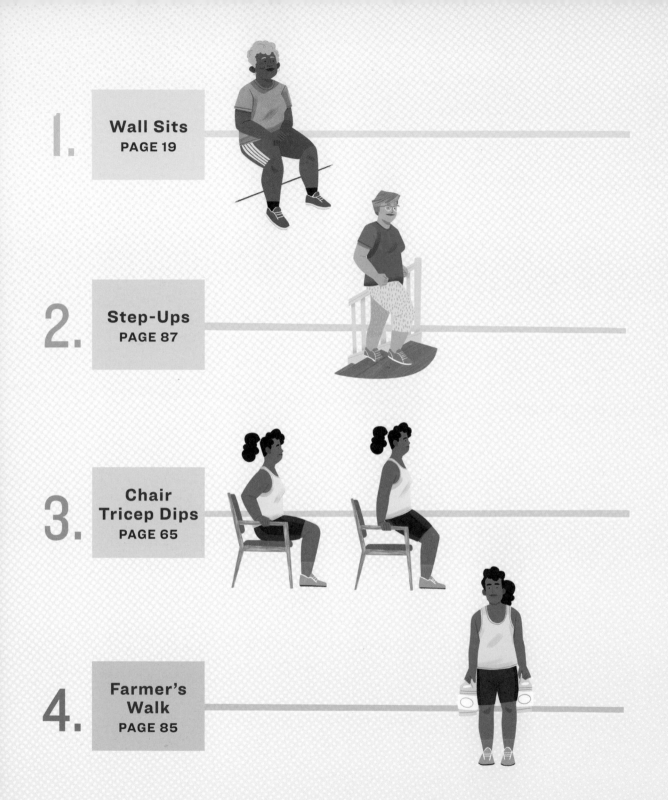

1. **Wall Sits**
PAGE 19

2. **Step-Ups**
PAGE 87

3. **Chair Tricep Dips**
PAGE 65

4. **Farmer's Walk**
PAGE 85

JET-SETTER

TARGETED BENEFITS: Bone Density, Endurance, Joint Health

If you embrace life's adventures, both near and far, this routine, designed for those who refuse to let age limit their travel aspirations, is for you. Travel requires strength to carry luggage, endurance to walk longer distances, and lower-body strength and agility to climb the stairs of ancient ruins. This routine has you covered with a combination of total body and bone building strengthening exercises and exercises that focus on improving joint health.

THE ROUTINE

1. **WALL SITS:** 8 to 12 repetitions for 2 or 3 sets

   30 to 60 seconds' rest in between sets

2. **STEP-UPS:** 8 to 10 repetitions for 2 or 3 sets

   30 to 60 seconds' rest in between sets

3. **CHAIR TRICEP DIPS:** 8 to 12 repetitions for 2 or 3 sets

   30 to 60 seconds' rest in between sets

4. **FARMER'S WALK:** 15 to 20 steps per set. Repeat for 2 or 3 sets

   30 to 60 seconds' rest in between sets

Remember: Chair Dips may be difficult if your armrests are too high. If so, use a pillow on the seat to raise you up a bit. Focus on keeping your grip strength strong during the Farmer's Walk and increase the weight so it's challenging. You can even use luggage for weights!

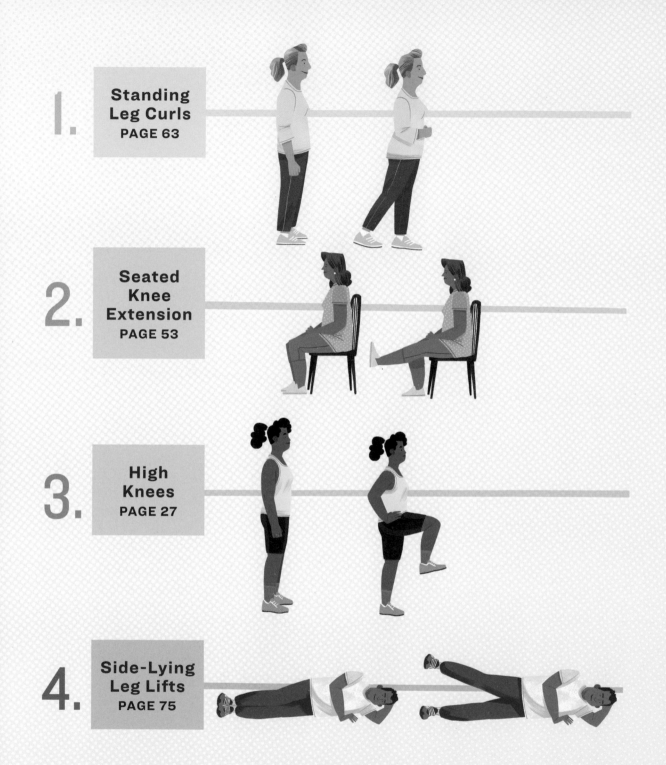

1. Standing
Leg Curls
PAGE 63

2. Seated
Knee
Extension
PAGE 53

3. High
Knees
PAGE 27

4. Side-Lying
Leg Lifts
PAGE 75

JOINT JUICE JIVE

TARGETED BENEFITS: Aches and Pains, Mobility

Don't let joint pain keep you from the things you love to do. Grease the wheels and ease the pain of achy hips and knees with this routine designed to reduce the aches and pains in your legs and improve lower-body strength and hip mobility. With a lower-body focus, this routine helps increase joint lubrication, promote overall joint health, and reduce pain-producing inflammation by strengthening the muscles supporting your hips and knees.

THE ROUTINE

1. **STANDING LEG CURLS:** 8 to 12 repetitions for 2 or 3 sets

   30 to 60 seconds' rest in between sets

2. **SEATED KNEE EXTENSION:** 8 to 12 repetitions for 2 or 3 sets

   30 to 60 seconds' rest in between sets

3. **HIGH KNEES:** 8 to 12 repetitions for 2 or 3 sets

   30 to 60 seconds' rest in between sets

4. **SIDE-LYING LEG LIFTS:** 8 to 12 repetitions for 2 or 3 sets

   30 to 60 seconds' rest in between sets

Remember: Increase the speed of the repetitions of the High Knees exercise as you feel stronger and try to challenge your balance by not holding on for support. On the Side-Lying Leg Lifts, keep the motion from your hips by not lifting your leg too high.

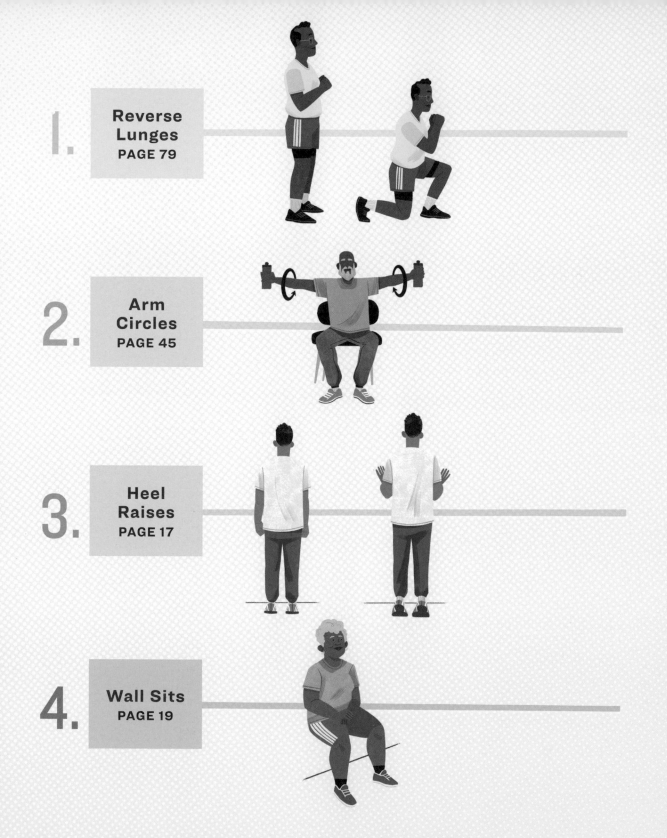

1. Reverse Lunges PAGE 79

2. Arm Circles PAGE 45

3. Heel Raises PAGE 17

4. Wall Sits PAGE 19

THE BOOGIE BOOSTER

TARGETED BENEFITS: Endurance, Metabolic Health

Do you love to dance? Designed to enhance your dancing abilities and maintain your youthful spirit, this routine focuses on key areas to help you shine on the dance floor. By incorporating exercises that improve hip strength and endurance, strengthen your ankles to stay light on your feet, and exercises that improve arm muscle endurance, you can ensure a lifetime of dancing.

THE ROUTINE

1. **REVERSE LUNGES:** 8 to 12 repetitions for 2 or 3 sets

   30 to 60 seconds' rest in between sets

2. **ARM CIRCLES:** 8 to 12 repetitions for 2 or 3 sets

   30 to 60 seconds' rest in between sets

3. **HEEL RAISES:** 8 to 12 repetitions for 2 or 3 sets

   30 to 60 seconds' rest in between sets

4. **WALL SITS:** 8 to 12 repetitions for 2 or 3 sets

   30 to 60 seconds' rest in between sets

Remember: Progress to single-leg Heel Raises as you gain strength. Using a smooth wall or an exercise ball behind your back will make the Wall Sits easier to do.

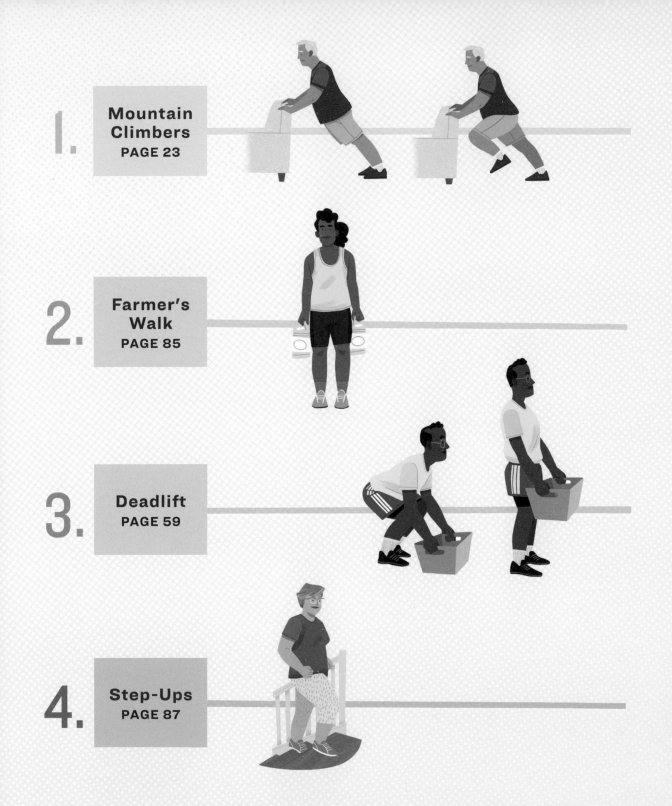

1. Mountain Climbers
PAGE 23

2. Farmer's Walk
PAGE 85

3. Deadlift
PAGE 59

4. Step-Ups
PAGE 87

PEAK PERFORMANCE

TARGETED BENEFITS: Bone Density, Endurance, Metabolic Health, Muscle Mass

Elevate your fitness and unleash your strength with this challenging routine. Not for the faint of heart, this routine is designed for those who have been exercising but want to go next level with their fitness. By engaging in higher-level exercises such as Deadlifts and Mountain Climbers, you'll supercharge your metabolism and promote efficient calorie burning to help you maintain a healthy weight.

THE ROUTINE

1. **MOUNTAIN CLIMBERS:** 8 to 12 repetitions for 2 or 3 sets

   30 to 60 seconds' rest in between sets

2. **FARMER'S WALK:** 15 to 20 steps per set. Repeat for 2 or 3 sets

   30 to 60 seconds' rest in between sets

3. **DEADLIFT:** 8 to 12 repetitions for 2 or 3 sets

   30 to 60 seconds' rest in between sets

4. **STEP-UPS:** 8 to 10 repetitions for 2 or 3 sets

   30 to 60 seconds' rest in between sets

Remember: To get an even better workout, reduce your rest time between sets to really get your heart pumping!

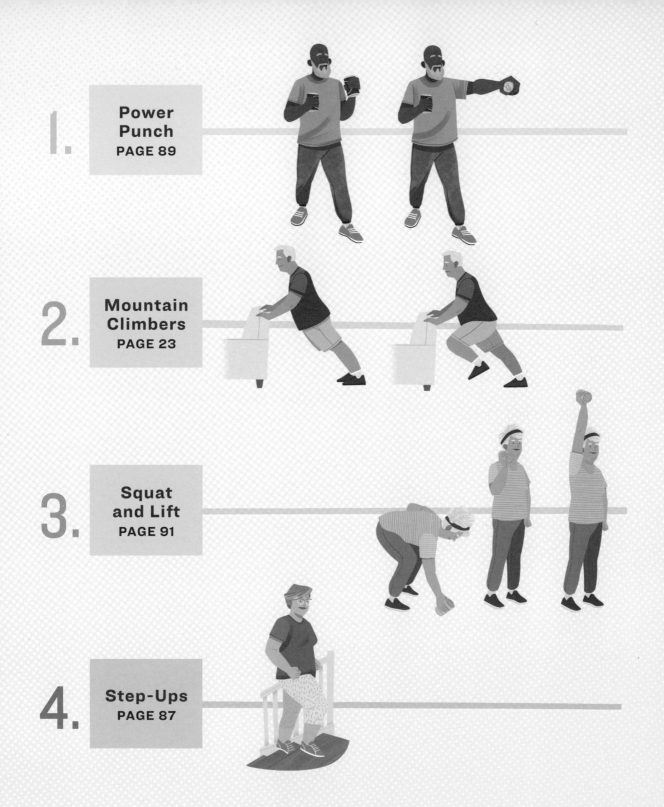

1. Power Punch
PAGE 89

2. Mountain Climbers
PAGE 23

3. Squat and Lift
PAGE 91

4. Step-Ups
PAGE 87

POWER PUMP

TARGETED BENEFITS: Balance, Bone Density, Joint Health Mobility

Punch, step, and climb your way to better health and fitness with this advanced routine designed for those who have already been exercising but want to take fitness to new heights. With a combination of power, agility, muscular endurance, and speed exercises, you will improve your stability and balance, help build bone density, and supercharge your aerobic fitness.

THE ROUTINE

1. **POWER PUNCH:** 8 to 10 repetitions for 2 or 3 sets

   30 to 60 seconds' rest in between sets

2. **MOUNTAIN CLIMBERS:** 8 to 12 repetitions for 2 or 3 sets

   30 to 60 seconds' rest in between sets

3. **SQUAT AND LIFT:** 6 to 10 repetitions for 2 or 3 sets

   30 to 60 seconds' rest in between sets

4. **STEP-UPS:** 8 to 12 repetitions for 2 or 3 sets

   30 to 60 seconds' rest in between sets

Remember: Shorten up the rest time in between sets to maximize your cardio fitness. To increase the power of your hips, you can try stepping up two stairs with the Step-Up exercise.

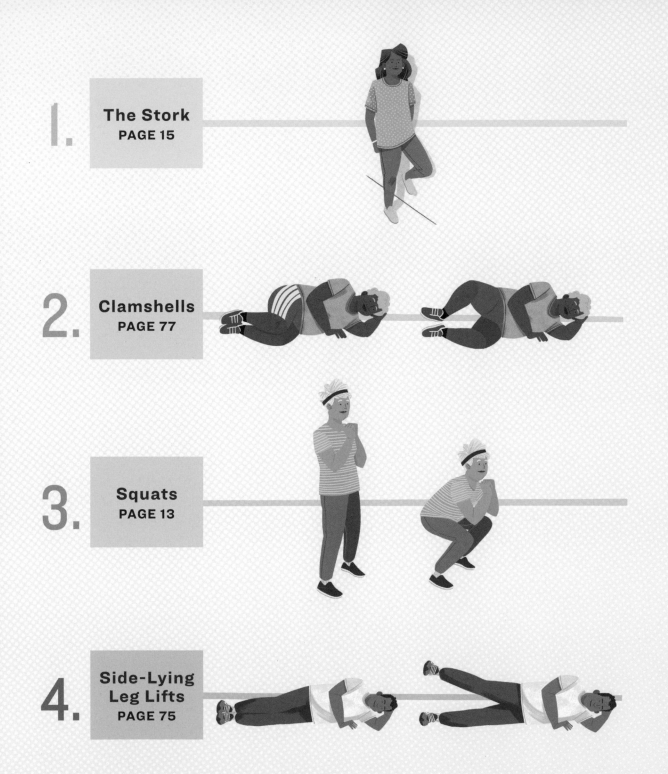

1. The Stork
PAGE 15

2. Clamshells
PAGE 77

3. Squats
PAGE 13

4. Side-Lying Leg Lifts
PAGE 75

KNEE PAIN KNOCKOUT

TARGETED BENEFITS: Aches and Pains, Joint Health, Mobility

Knee pain can make daily activities, such as walking and climbing steps, difficult and painful, resulting in a loss of independence and function. But kick knee pain to the curb with this routine designed to reduce knee pain and improve strength and function of your knees. Knee pain often stems from weakness in the hips and lower legs. This routine tackles this issue head-on by targeting and strengthening your hips and lower legs with a combination of functional exercises like Squats and isolated muscle strengthening exercises like Heel Raises.

THE ROUTINE

I. **THE STORK:** Hold for 10 to 15 seconds per set. Repeat for 2 or 3 sets

   30 to 60 seconds' rest in between sets

2. **CLAMSHELLS:** 8 to 12 repetitions for 2 or 3 sets

   30 to 60 seconds' rest in between sets

3. **SQUATS:** 8 to 12 repetitions for 2 or 3 sets

   30 to 60 seconds' rest in between sets

4. **SIDE-LYING LEG LIFTS:** 8 to 12 repetitions for 2 or 3 sets

   30 to 60 seconds' rest in between sets

Remember: Make your hips and core really work by pushing as hard as you can with the Stork exercise and increase your hold times as you get stronger. For Heel Raises, use just a single leg to really challenge your strength.

References

Brown, Lee E., and Vance A. Ferrigno. *Training for Speed, Agility, and Quickness*. Champaign, IL: Human Kinetics, 2015.

Reid, Kieran F., Kimberly I. Martin, Gheorghe Doros, David J. Clark, Cynthia Hau, Carolynn Patten, Edward M. Phillips, et al. "Comparative Effects of Light or Heavy Resistance Power Training for Improving Lower Extremity Power and Physical Performance in Mobility-Limited Older Adults." *The Journals of Gerontology: Series A* 70, no. 3 (2015): 372–78. doi:10.1093/gerona/glu156.

Rippetoe, Mark, Andy Baker, and Stephani Elizabeth Bradford. *Practical Programming for Strength Training*. Wichita Falls, TX: The Aasgaard Company, 2017.

Rippetoe, Mark, and Stephani Elizabeth Bradford. *Starting Strength: Basic Barbell Training*. Wichita Falls, TX: The Aasgaard Company, 2017.

Rowe, John W., MD, and Robert L. Kahn, PhD. *Successful Aging*. New York: Pantheon Books, 1998.

Waehner, Paige. *Strength Training for Seniors: Increase Your Balance, Stability, and Stamina to Rewind the Aging Process*. New York: Skyhorse Publishing, 2020.

Index

Notes

ABOUT THE AUTHOR

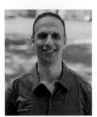 **Ed Deboo** is a physical therapist with over twenty-nine years of clinical experience. He is co-owner of Integrative Physical Therapy in Bellingham, Washington. Ed graduated from Western Washington University with a degree in exercise science and holds a master of science degree in physical therapy from Des Moines University.

Ed is also a Level 1–certified sports coach and is BoneFit USA certified to work with clients with low bone density. With a passion for health and fitness, he shares exercise and self-care tips on his YouTube channel, *Front Row with Ed and Elizabeth*.